Why are you pretending to be normal?

DR PHIL FRIEND OBE AND DAVE REES

This edition first published in 2013
by Friend and Rees Publishing.

© Phil Friend and Dave Rees.

All rights reserved. No part of this
publication may be reproduced or
transmitted in any form or by any
means electronic or mechanical,
including photocopying, recording
or any information storage
and retrieval system, without
permission in writing from the
publishers.

British Library Cataloguing in
Publication Data
A catalogue record for this book is
available from the British Library.

ISBN: 978-0-9575999-0-1
10 9 8 7 6 5 4 3 2 1

Printed and bound by Gemini Press

	Foreword	4
1	Dawn	6
2	George	12
3	Angela	36
4	Jan	58
5	Paul	88
6	Me	116
7	You	124

Foreword
Baroness Tanni Grey-Thompson DBE

This book masterfully guides the reader to an understanding of the importance of the social model of disability and will be extremely useful to a wide audience who want to learn and understand about the impact language has on people's lives.

This book goes beyond telling people the 'right' words to use, as the personalisation of Chris' journey helps the reader understand the relationship between language and attitude in a skillful way. With each chapter, as you learn a little more about the journey, the understanding of the issues builds.

Discovering the social model of disability was a light bulb moment for me. It helped me put in to context what being a wheelchair user would mean. It was easy to understand that if physical access was improved then my life would be easier too.

But it took a little bit longer to learn that attitudinal change was important as well, both mine and other peoples. Once you start to understand that 'language is the dress of thought', then improving your understanding as well as that of others becomes paramount.

If other people understood more about my needs and felt able to ask me, instead of making assumptions (which were quite often the wrong ones) then my life would dramatically improve.

But I learnt that a responsibility also fell on me. I could quite often get frustrated with how I was treated, but I learnt that if I had a better understanding of not just what to ask for, but the way in which to explain my impairment, then that could also have a significant impact on how I was treated.

Using the story of Chris, it becomes really clear how every disabled person can have a positive impact on the wider understanding of disability and impairment.

I hope that you will enjoy this book as much as I did.

1 Dawn

Something happened that day that radically changed my approach to life forever.

This 'something' started with a question of just seven words. It led me to meet some fascinating people who were very ordinary but looked at life in an extraordinary way. As a result of meeting them, I recognised things about myself that I had never considered before and because I had never considered them, I had been at risk of not realising anything like my true potential.

But before I tell you about my journey and what I learnt from meeting these people, you need to know something else.

My name is Chris and I am part of an interesting club.

The majority of people in the world are born without a disability and I was one of these. However, I will now be one of the majority of people in the world who will die with one, having 'acquired' my disability during my adult life. I did not want it, I never asked for it but disability came calling anyway.

It is important for my story that you know this. I feel compelled to share the lessons I have learnt that have helped me and could help you, not just to cope with your disability, but to actually manage it and its impact.

On the day that began my change in thinking, I was on a course with a group of people, some of whom I knew, but the majority of whom I had never met before. Much of what was being taught was new to me but there was some information and ideas that I had already seen before. I found myself sitting next to a lady called Dawn. At various intervals throughout the day the course trainer asked us to discuss a number of different topics with the person next to us and so I was paired up with Dawn.

During one of the group sessions several contributors started talking about disability. This made me feel quite uncomfortable as I knew one of the course participants was aware that I was disabled and I hoped that they did not bring up the fact during the conversation.

At the end of the course I was walking out of the training room with Dawn who kindly commented that she had enjoyed the conversations we'd had in our pairing and that she had learnt a lot from them.

We carried on talking about other aspects from the day for about ten minutes before she asked me **that** question.

'I understand that you're disabled,' she said.

Embarrassed and taken aback by her directness, I replied that I was.

'So why are you pretending to be normal?'

Why are you pretending to be normal

I was stunned. Astounded! I didn't know what to say, where to look or what to do next. What did she mean? Who the hell did she think she was? How dare she say something like that to me! What business was it of hers? I groped around for some words and eventually muttered, 'What exactly do you mean?'

Dawn looked me straight in the eye and said confidently, 'I'm really not trying to be rude or anything like that I assure you. It's just that I heard from one of the course participants that you're disabled and yet you behave and act as if you're not. I find that really very interesting.'

Dawn's simple but profound question began a transformation in me. It was this question that led me to meet a series of people. And it was these people who helped me to reposition myself and rethink my disability and the impact it has on me and those around me.

Once I'd collected my thoughts and got past my initial shock, I shared with Dawn the fact that I was having some difficulty 'coming to terms' with my disability. Dawn said she knew and worked with people who could help me with this if I was willing to meet them. She explained that they would not help me to 'come to terms' with my impairment, but actually help me to learn to live with it which was a very big difference and one that I didn't fully understand at that time.

Despite serious misgivings on my part, we exchanged contact details and Dawn said that if I wanted, she would arrange some meetings for me over the following couple of weeks with four of her associates. Somewhat apprehensive, but intrigued, I agreed. True to her word Dawn contacted me the next day with details of the meetings.

What follows is the story of the concepts that Dawn's four colleagues helped me to learn, and the thoughts they shared that helped me to rethink my attitude towards my disability. They also helped me to unlearn some of the fundamental ideas that had guided, influenced and in fact limited me for so long.

The first meeting was with a chap called George.

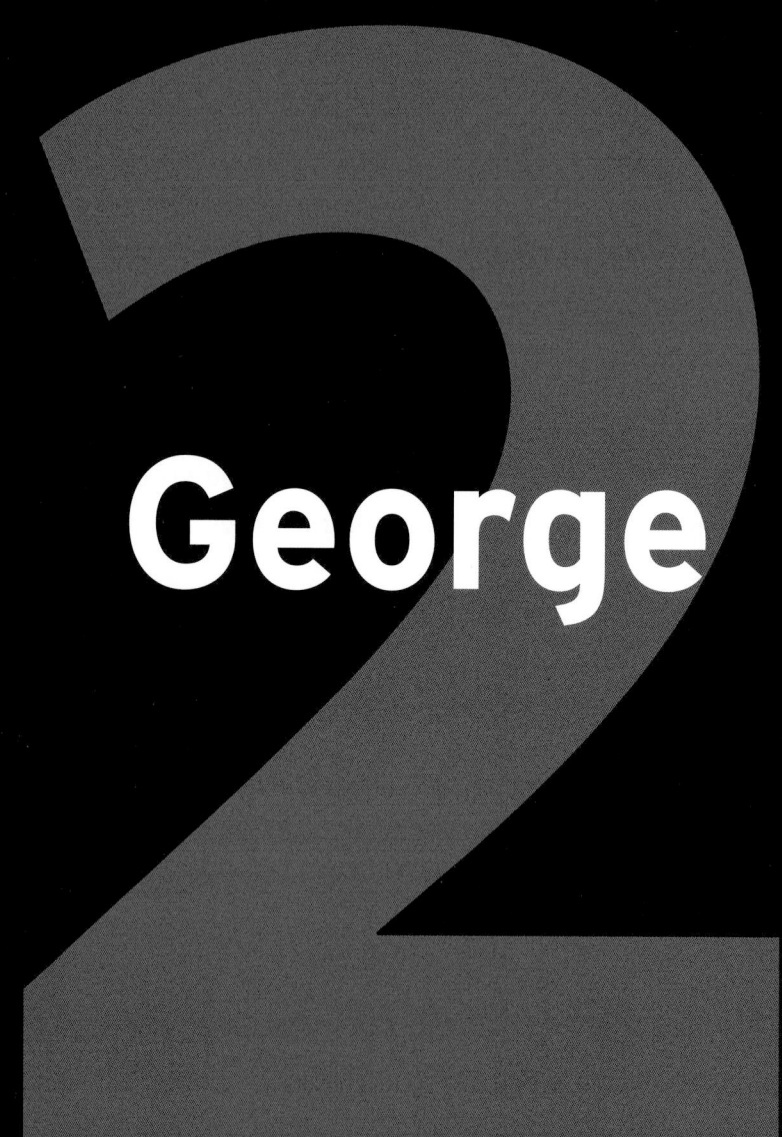

George lived in a bungalow situated in a quiet cul-de-sac. After I had rung the door bell, the door opened to reveal a tall, casually dressed man with a warm smile and a firm handshake. After we'd introduced ourselves he beckoned me in enthusiastically.

'Come through. Please sit down. Would you like a drink?' he enquired as he gestured towards a leather sofa across the back wall of his elegant lounge.

'That would be very nice. Coffee please – just milk and no sugar,' I replied.

'Really good to meet you Chris,' continued George. 'Dawn told me to expect you. An interesting woman don't you think? Now let's get that coffee organised.'

While George made the coffee, I reflected on the purpose of my visit. I was surprised at how anxious I was feeling and wondered how I should start such a sensitive conversation about disability with a complete stranger. I knew that I wanted to make the most of the discussion with him but was wary of talking about my personal situation with someone whom I had only just met. I was also puzzled because Dawn had said that George was disabled and yet I couldn't see anything obviously 'wrong' with him.

With that thought in mind, I decided that I should take the initiative and drive the agenda. Taking a deep breath, I plunged in.

'It's really good of you to spare the time to see me George. Dawn said that you might share your knowledge of disability with me and that it would help me to manage my disability more effectively.' Then, a little more nervously, I added, 'Perhaps you could start by telling me what's wrong with you?'

George's answer took me by surprise.

'There's nothing wrong with me!' he exclaimed. 'What's wrong with you?'

Oops! Not an encouraging start. I tried frantically to rephrase the question.

'Sorry. I didn't mean to...' I stammered, fidgeting about uncomfortably on the sofa. 'What I meant was what's the matter with you? What's your disability?' I felt incredibly stupid and embarrassed. What was I doing asking such a personal question so soon? We'd only just met. Had I offended George before our conversation had even really begun?

George looked at me inquisitively and then slowly smiled.

'You need to learn a very important principle if you're really going to manage your disability effectively,' he said in a much more friendly tone.

'Basically,' he continued, 'I don't have a disability.'

'Oh. I'm sorry. I thought from my conversation with Dawn that you were disabled and that's why I should talk with you.'

I suddenly felt disappointed. I wanted to make sense of what had happened to me and felt a little cheated that what had seemed like an opportunity may actually have been a waste of my time.

'The first thing to really understand,' continued George confidently, 'is that I don't have a disability. I actually have what is termed 'an impairment'. To be more accurate it's a hearing impairment. It happened when I was a teenager. I'm fairly sure that it can't be fixed and as a result I'm never going to have so-called normal hearing again.'

I was confused and asked, 'Does it really matter what you call it? An impairment? A disability? Surely it's all the same thing isn't it?'

'Oh, but it does matter!' George said firmly. 'You see, neither of us can cure my impairment but we can both do something about my disability. I have a hearing impairment as I said. My impairment is a hearing loss. But I'm only disabled when people turn away from me when they are talking or they cover their mouth with their hand so I can't lip read. I'm disabled when my manager runs a meeting where everybody can talk at once and I can't work out or focus on who's talking and as a result I miss a lot of what people are saying.'

'Oh you're just playing around with words,' I said rather condescendingly. 'It's just splitting hairs; people don't really make that sort of distinction between whether something is an impairment or a disability.' I wanted to push George into providing some kind of evidence that would convince me this wasn't just him being politically correct.

Without hesitating George continued, 'I'm not a fan of the word 'impairment' to be honest. I wish I could find a better word. But Chris isn't there a difference between what I have, my hearing loss, and what I am able to do as result of having that condition? I have what I have. But other factors and other people get in the way of me being able to perform to my full potential. If you turn around to look at that photograph on the wall behind you I can't see what your lips are doing and so I can't hear what you're saying. You've disabled me! Other people do that all the time. They disable me. And if all I do is just moan about it or put up with it, I am in fact disabling myself as I am focusing on the 'dis' of disability rather than the 'ability'.'

> Do I focus on my **'dis'** or my **'ability'**?

I began to understand what George was saying. This wasn't political correctness but was about using language more precisely. Ironically he was the one with the hearing loss and yet I was only now hearing what he was saying. I was intrigued and impressed. What a simple but powerful message.

'So are you saying that I'm only disabled if I let others disable me?'

'Exactly! Someone in a wheelchair is disabled because there isn't a ramp to get into the building. Someone who is partially sighted is disabled because they are given a document with a print size that's too small for them to

> **I have an impairment not a disability.**

read. Disability is often the outcome of an impairment and it's our own or society's attitude that disables us.'

George could tell by looking at me that I had got the message.

I have an impairment not a disability.

I can't do much about my impairment, but I can do a lot about my disability!

'What you need to realise Chris is that there's nothing 'wrong' with you,' he continued. 'There's nothing 'the matter' with you. There's nothing 'odd' about you. You've just acquired an impairment. I'm sure it's distressing, confusing and possibly painful. It's also incredibly frustrating because the impairment stops you doing some of the things that you did before you had it and I'm sure you would rather not have it. But at the end of the day if you think there's something 'wrong' with you, then you will think, behave and talk from that perspective. Everyone else will then pick up on those signals and start to think the same. As a result, there is a real danger that you will see yourself as worse than other people who are non-disabled.'

> I can't do much about my impairment, **but I can do a lot about my disability!**

'Why don't you call them able-bodied?' I asked.

'Able-bodied suggests that they are somehow better than me,' George responded. 'To refer to others as non-disabled seems to equalise the position. It is also true to say that someone could have an impairment such as dyslexia but be physically 'able-bodied' so the term non-disabled describes those without impairments more accurately. A bit confusing but I hope you see what I mean?'

I was fascinated by this very different perspective, which became clearer the more we talked. I had never considered things this way before and I asked George whether the language we used really mattered that much.

He said he believed it is language that has been disabling us for years because it has influenced how we and other people view disability. They see the 'dis' – what you can't do – rather than what you can. George explained that he had a good job, could cook really well, that he was a fast runner, a very good tennis player, a loving husband, a devoted parent with two fantastic kids and was on the committee of some local organisations. But none of these really registered in people's perception of his disability. He queried whether the most interesting thing about him was his impairment or the fact that he is a sports fan, a parent and a supportive work colleague? He jokingly said that he was also a vegetarian and that on occasions he gets better service and greater understanding for that than he does for being disabled – and vegetarians don't have as many legal rights! When people see him as a 'disabled' person they see him as unable to do certain things as well as they can.

'So what you're saying is that I need to use the right words, the right language. How would you define the right language? Sounds like we're back to political correctness!'

'Absolutely not!' George exclaimed. 'This isn't about trivialising the issue. Language defines us all. We don't refer to 'cripples' or 'invalids' any more because the terms are now seen to be derogatory and demeaning. Nothing trivial about that. Let me give you an example of what I mean.'

George got up and walked across to the window. Looking out, and pausing for a moment, he continued. 'I recently met an old friend, Peter, who I hadn't seen for some time. He told me that he had been "suffering with a bad back". Well I'm sure his back was very painful and as far as Peter was concerned the description is pretty accurate. But as soon as he used the word 'suffering' do you know what that made me feel?'

George didn't wait for my answer.

'Well, I'll tell you,' he continued. 'I felt sorry for him. I felt pity. I felt sympathy. I asked him whether he wanted me to feel pity and sympathy for him and he got pretty irritated and said, 'No way'. I suggested that in order to stop others feeling like that he needed to change the way he described his impairment. He was disabling himself with the language he was using and so now he says that he has back pain or a painful back and then goes on to describe what he needs to manage it as productively as possible. Far better, wouldn't you say?'

I really understood what George was saying and while I collected my thoughts I suggested that you reap what you sow.

'Exactly,' said George. 'If I was Peter's manager, think of the impact if I continually felt sorry for him. Most of my interactions with him would be driven by my feelings of pity and sympathy. In fact I may choose to protect Peter from further pain by not giving him additional work that he actually wants to do. Or I may avoid him altogether because I don't know how to deal with him. Either way his chances of promotion must surely be seriously jeopardised. I just see him 'suffering' from a bad back. I don't see his potential because of the way he views and describes himself.'

George returned to his armchair. 'As someone once said, "Are you part of the problem or part of the solution?" The answer is both. You need to change the way you describe yourself and your impairment and you will get a different response. If you see your impairment as a negative how do you convince others that it can be a positive?'

'I see your point. I really do,' I said enthusiastically. 'But I think you've hit on another problem there. To be honest on most occasions I don't really describe my disability, I mean my impairment. And when I do, I see it as a negative and so will everyone else. I get that.'

'You have to position all this properly,' continued George. 'Have you ever been in a situation where you have lost someone close to you?'

I replied that I had lost two friends a few years ago to cancer.

'Well obviously I'm sorry to hear about that,' said George sympathetically. 'If you know anything about the way we grieve or deal with bereavement, then you'll remember some of the emotions you went through after their deaths.'

George went on to explain the different emotions that people experience during the grieving process and I recognised each stage as if he were talking directly about me. I remembered the first emotions of shock and denial that I felt when I heard that my friends had died. I also remembered that initially I didn't believe the news and that I needed to be told a number of times before it sunk in. These feelings were followed by a whole host of emotions such as anger, blame, guilt, frustration and anxiety. I had accepted that my friends were dead but I still had this huge variety of emotions about how it had all happened, how unfair it was and how I was going to cope without them. I also knew that their families had received some counselling to help them to better deal with this continuous cycle of emotions so that they could distance themselves more and more from the pain of their loss. George explained that this counselling was about helping people to work through this cycle of emotions until they started to feel more positive. Of course they were still grieving but they also felt how privileged they were to have known the people who had died. It is only then they really started to create that distance between themselves and the pain.

'Well acquiring an impairment is very similar,' continued George. 'When you become disabled you also have to go through that same cycle of emotions because you have lost something, whether it's something physical – because you can no longer walk or move other parts of your body – or whether it's the loss of independence or anything else. It is also the loss of the person you used to be, and the feeling that you can no longer be the person you were before you got this. Therefore you go through the same emotions of shock, denial, anger, frustration and all the other stages of grief until you come to accept it – if you ever do!'

I knew exactly what George meant and realised that I could honestly say I had not yet come to terms with my disability. I was one of the many people who were now members of the disability club but who still considered life from a non-disabled viewpoint.

I vividly remembered the moment when I learnt the truth about my impairment and my feelings of shock. I then went into denial: I wanted to pretend it was all a dream, or a nightmare. There must be a cure or there has been a terrible mistake with the diagnosis! That was my defence mechanism kicking in – it will never happen to me. Then followed some form of acceptance that I was now disabled but all those feelings of anger, blame, guilt and frustration all kept revisiting me as I struggled to come to terms with what the future held for me. I realised that I was still feeling these emotions. I was trying to hide my impairment and pretend it was not there but actually it was now a part of me. It was not only the language that I was using with others that had to be changed but also the conversations I was having with myself. That was where I needed to start.

I could feel myself becoming quite emotional and close to tears. George waited patiently while I tried to make sense of my feelings. 'If this didn't matter,' he said, 'you wouldn't be feeling so strongly about it.'

Although embarrassed to have almost wept in front of a total stranger, I somehow felt as if I had known George for years because he understood. Understanding the impact of disability is something that people without a disability often find difficult to do.

It doesn't matter what the impairment is, we all go through the same emotional curve.

After a bit of nose blowing and a second cup of coffee, I settled and asked George whether I should tell people about my impairment and if so when. He thought about the question and said that I should tell people about my impairment when it was appropriate. This left me a little confused, but before I could launch into another series of questions George suggested that we should bring our conversation to a close for the day and, before I met Dawn's next associate, Angela, I should think about these questions:

- ▶▶ Why don't you discuss your impairment?
- ▶▶ When you don't discuss it, why not?
- ▶▶ When you do discuss it, why?
- ▶▶ How do you discuss it?

I thanked George for his kindness and for sparing the time to meet me. I told him that our conversation had really helped me focus on the importance of language and he had also helped me to begin the process of accepting my impairment. As I made my way down the street, I felt a sense of renewed energy and determination and a real desire to begin the next stage of my journey.

Be aware of your language.

Be conscious of how you describe yourself and your impairment.

Otherwise you could be **disabling yourself!**

Why don't you talk about your impairment?

When you don't discuss it, **why not**?

When you do discuss it, **why**?

How do you discuss it?

Reflecting on my conversation with George, I realised that I needed to talk to other people in a way that helped them to treat me as I wanted to be treated and how I deserved to be treated. I also needed to talk to myself in a much more positive way. George had said something else which I thought was very profound as we finished our conversation. He said, 'I am who I am as a result of my disability, not in spite of it. It helps to shape and influence the person I am.'

I was really looking forward to meeting my next contact Angela in a few days' time to continue challenging my thinking.

However before that I was keen to make the most of my newfound knowledge. I found myself taking extra care to listen closely to the words that people used and I kept asking myself what sort of impact these people had on me as a result of their language.

When I greeted people and asked them how they were, I noticed the subtle yet different effect it had on me when one replied, 'not bad' whereas another replied, 'really good thanks'. I also started to notice their differing tones of voice and felt their enthusiasm when they were upbeat and their lack of passion and commitment when their message was conveyed with no energy.

When I met or saw disabled people talking about themselves on television, in newspaper articles and books they would often describe themselves as 'suffering' just as George had suggested. I realised the effect it had on me in the main was negative or invoked pity or sympathy. Other people were describing themselves as having a 'hearing defect', as being 'wheelchair-bound', as having a 'funny walk' or being a 'stroke victim' and I analysed the effect that these descriptions had on me. In each case, I tended to feel sorrow and pity and saw them somehow diminished and damaged as people. I saw the problem rather than the person – the 'dis' rather than the 'ability'.

On one television programme I watched, a person described himself as 'a diabetic'. I was really struck by the idea that he saw himself as a condition first and a person second. Clearly diabetes is a serious health condition and needs to be managed carefully but surely you are a person who has the condition rather than being it! It seemed to me that saying you are someone who has diabetes is preferable, more accurate and more positive.

Immersed in my thoughts, discussions began with my

partner and interestingly we explored what the benefits of having a condition like diabetes might be. To manage it well, you'd certainly have to be creative; you'd need to develop good problem solving skills very quickly; you would need to be resilient and determined and develop strong time management skills. All of these potentially positive attributes are lost when a person describes themselves as a 'diabetic', emphasising the 'dis' rather than the 'ability'. Better to have said, 'I have this condition which means that

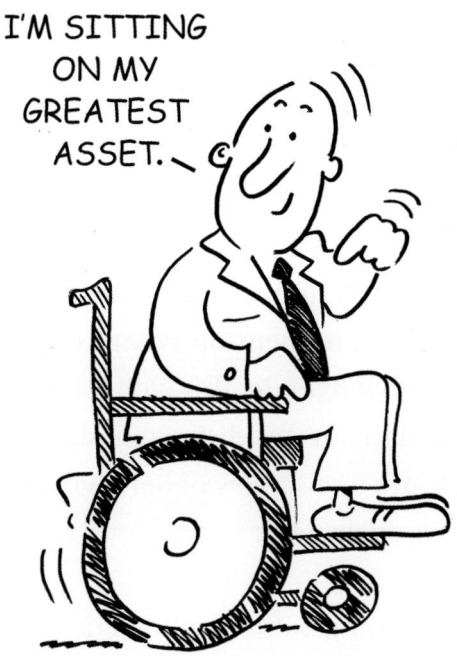

I apply this particular set of skills every day of my life'. We also concluded that people should use positive statements to describe themselves for example saying that they have a 'memorable walk' rather than a 'funny walk'; subtle repositioning but with a very different impact.

Another way of putting this for example is to describe someone as 'having a problem' rather than 'being a problem'.

On reflection, I could see that the way in which I previously described my own situation was about being a problem rather than having a problem to deal with. I now understood my choice of words when talking about my impairment to others had a negative or positive effect. In other words, it wasn't difficult for me to disable myself.

I knew that it was important when in conversations with myself, or others, to focus on what I could do, rather than what I could no longer do; this would help me to emphasise my ability and to put the 'dis' to one side. It would also help me through my own cycles of bereavement even though I still had my impairment.

Before others could value me, I needed to value myself.

This was all learning that I was keen to share with Angela when I kept my appointment with her later that day.

Angela 3

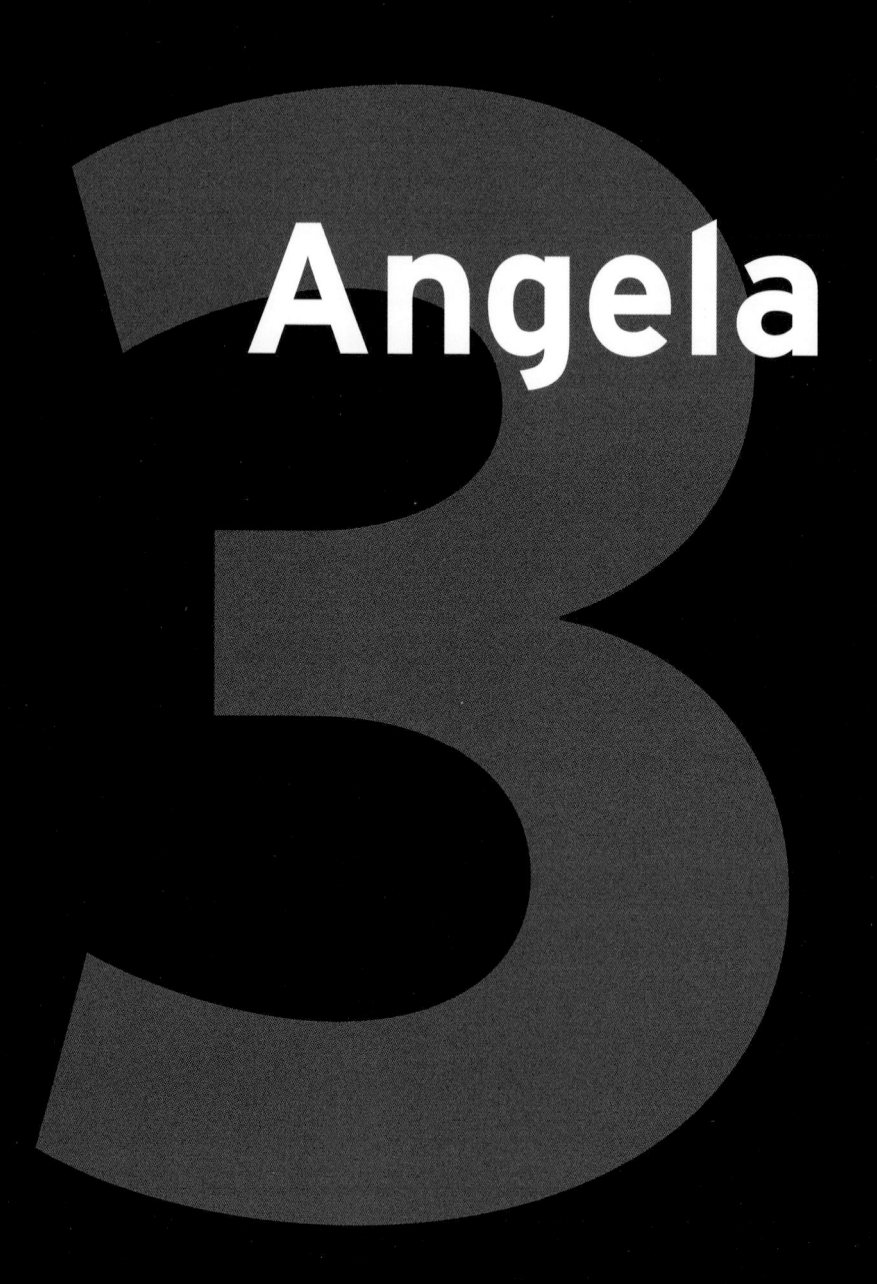

Like George, Angela gave me a warm welcome. She was taller than me, dressed casually and had an infectious grin. She took me through to her kitchen and offered me a seat and a drink. The comfortable kitchen was clearly used as a family room and furnished in a farmhouse style. At one end of the room was a large dresser, which displayed all sorts of antique jugs and plates. I took a seat opposite at a large round table while Angela made us both a drink and asked about my journey and whether I'd found the house easily. She eventually joined me at the table and I felt relaxed and keen to show her that I really had mastered George's first lessons.

'I've been really looking forward to meeting you Angela. It's so good of you to spare the time. I learned so much from George. During my time with him we focussed on how the language we use can actually disable us more.'

She readily agreed. 'Oh George! He's got such a great outlook on life hasn't he? He is of course quite right about the language we use. I remember asking him once over a meal, "Can you tell me how deaf you are?" Do you know what he said? "How hearing are you?" Brilliant reply, don't you think?'

I laughed at the unexpected nature of the response. I could see myself challenging my assumption that we tend to view people's impairments from the perspective of everyone being 100% ok but why should we? I was keen to learn more but wanted to make sure that I didn't put my foot in it at the start of the conversation with Angela as I so nearly had with George.

I chose my words really carefully especially as, like George, Angela did not have an obvious impairment. 'So forgive me for asking, but what's your impairment Angela? I'm guessing that it's a hidden impairment as it's not very obvious.'

'I can see that George has changed your thinking about the words you need to use,' said Angela with a broad smile, 'although I feel that you still need a little more practice! You see my impairment isn't 'hidden', it's just not visible to you.'

'Well when I say 'hidden' I mean that I can't see it. Same thing really.'

'Is 'hidden' really the same as 'not visible' Chris? Examine the language and the meaning of the words? Don't you see the difference?'

I confessed that I didn't.

'If it were 'hidden' then that suggests that I'm deliberately keeping it from you. That kind of indicates that I am ashamed or uncomfortable or that I haven't learned how to manage the impairment or learned how to live with it. You might then interpret this as me trying to hide my impairment or understand it to be a taboo subject to be avoided at all costs. Describing the impairment as 'not visible' is quite different. You see me as a human being, equal to you, who just happens to have issues that I am dealing with. Using a term like 'not visible' might also suggest that you just haven't noticed.'

Is your impairment

'hidden'

or just

'not visible'?

I was disappointed with myself. I thought that I'd really cracked the language issue. Yet here was another valuable lesson and one that I really needed to grasp.

Ever since I had become disabled, or perhaps better put, ever since I 'acquired my impairment', I had been trying to hide it: from my family and friends, from anyone I met and from myself! I reflected on the energy that this approach was taking out of me unnecessarily. Why do we hide our impairments? How much energy do we needlessly waste trying to conceal them? What purpose does that actually serve?

I had only been with Angela for a short while but I was already feeling more enlightened.

Angela went on to explain a concept which she described as 'appropriate sharing'. Disability sometimes forces us to go public about things we would prefer to keep private. The concept of appropriate sharing focuses on how and when we should discuss our impairment with others and what it means for us. Several thoughts hit me at once. Do we need to share it? Couldn't we just keep it to ourselves? The idea of declaring or disclosing something has more to do with tax collection or an application for a passport, surely?

Angela and I agreed that we'd both met people who as soon as they introduced themselves also mentioned their disability. That seemed to be about sharing information too early. Why did they share it so readily and what was the point? Then there was the other end of the spectrum where people never told you what their impairment was when actually it would have been helpful for all concerned to mention it. Having a painful back, which limits mobility, is worth sharing if the plan is to go for a long walk. Reluctance to share important information could be linked to not wanting to admit that there is an issue – the denial stage of George's bereavement process, or not wanting to cause a fuss, or a fear that the information might be abused. Whatever the reason, does keeping quiet actually help?

I found it intriguing to reflect on how little I talked about my impairment and its impact to my colleagues at work. Was I trying to be brave and just get on with things? Maybe I was trying to still be the person I was before I acquired my impairment? On the other hand I wondered whether I was going on about it too much with my partner and close family to the point where they were getting bored with it and with me. With one group of people I was keeping it hidden and with others I was using it as an excuse.

I then recalled that an ex-colleague of mine had mentioned their non-visible impairment to someone at work in confidence, but that the person to whom it had been divulged had not kept the information private. This single incident had left such an impression on my colleague that from then on they decided not to share such information ever again. It was such a shame that because of one incident, my colleague then treated everyone with suspicion. I now realise he limited the assistance that might have been available to him and therefore became less effective at work as a result.

> Do I share my impairment **too early** or **not at all**?

> When should I discuss it **appropriately**?

I turned to Angela and said, 'Just now you used the phrase that someone had not "learned how to live with" rather than "come to terms with" their impairment. That was something Dawn mentioned to me when I met her. Is there a difference between the two phrases?'

'I believe so yes,' replied Angela as she settled back in her chair. 'Coming to terms' with your impairment seems a more negative statement than 'learning to live with it'. 'Coming to terms' suggests that you are coping with it whereas 'learning to live with it' is much more positive and suggests you're on top of it, you're managing it.'

Yet another example, I thought to myself, of the importance of language and of my need to make further progress in order to get my situation fully into perspective.

I was now really keen to hear what Angela had to share with me.

'Do you or any of your family and friends have children?' asked Angela casually.

I was a little surprised by the change of direction. I said that I didn't but that my sister had a lovely daughter called Rachel.

'Was Rachel born before you acquired your impairment?' asked Angela.

I replied that she was.

'When you heard the news of her birth what were the first questions you asked?'

I told her that I couldn't remember the precise details but that I must have commented that it was fantastic news, or something like that.

'So think about the questions you probably asked,' pressed Angela.

'Well if I remember rightly I heard that Laura had had her baby and then I firstly asked whether it was a boy or a girl.' I tried desperately to remember specifics of the moment but all I really remembered was the joy of hearing the news.

'That's usually the first question,' stated Angela. 'What was your second question?'

'I guess it was something like "is Laura ok? Is the baby all right?" I replied trying to drag the detail from my memory.

Angela nodded thoughtfully. 'That last question is an interesting one don't you think?' What does "is the baby all right" really mean?'

I hesitated; 'Err, well I suppose it's about whether or not there's anything wrong with it.'

As soon as I mentioned the word 'wrong' I began to see where Angela was going. I nearly shouted the phrase again as if in a eureka moment. 'Is there anything wrong with it? In other words 'is it normal?'

Angela was nodding at me, obviously pleased that I had seen what she was driving at. She then asked, 'What drove that question?'

'Well I obviously want the baby to be normal, to be healthy. Everyone does surely?'

'But you told me that one of George's principles was about the fact that there is nothing 'wrong' with you despite your condition. Well surely, if there's nothing wrong with you, doesn't that mean you are, as you put it, 'normal'?'

I suggested to Angela that there were a number of reasons

for me asking that question. Like most other people I wanted the child to live as normal a life as possible and was anxious that if the baby was disabled that it might not be able to do that. Everyone wants to fit in surely. It was also about people being able to take advantage of all the opportunities that might come their way.

Angela shared with me that when she had given birth to her three children she had been asked by lots of people who knew about her condition whether the children had been born disabled too. Why should people assume that just because she had an impairment then her children would too? Quite an assumption.

She continued by saying that since human beings have roamed this planet there have been people with impairments. In the early days of mankind if someone had an impairment that probably meant they could not see food or hear the approach of a hunter or be able enough to run away from danger. Having an impairment was an issue and nature dealt with it. The slowest got eaten and if you stayed behind to help the slowest you got eaten too. It has been part of the human story forever and history is full of examples of how our ancestors left the weak, the old, the injured and the disabled behind to die. Throughout time disabled people have been an 'easy target' for all manner of ill treatment, neglect or abuse and the subject has often invoked fear and sometimes sympathy. In more modern times we have actually been 'creating' more disabled people. Better sanitation, better housing and plentiful food has meant that the so-called weak survive for longer. However, in a society based around agriculture, it mattered less that people were blind. They could still follow a horse ploughing the fields as the horse was doing the 'seeing'. It is interesting to note that blind people became more disabled as a result of the Industrial Revolution, as getting to the factory and coping with the tasks inside it were more difficult. Similarly, groups of people with some learning impairments can experience real disadvantage as we become ever more dependent upon computing skills.

'I guess what I'm saying,' concluded Angela, 'is that we have always had people around who had some form of physical or mental impairment but as we have evolved we have disabled more and more of them.'

I found myself intrigued and fascinated by this historical perspective on disability. Before I could really get a handle on what she was saying Angela focused on the main point of our discussion.

'For me it all centres on this idea of being normal,' she said. 'But here is the crunch question: what's your definition of 'normal'?'

I suddenly felt somewhat uncomfortable as I reflected on my niece. What would I have done if I had been told she was not all right and that she had some sort of impairment? Would it have made a difference to the love I had for her at the moment of her birth and ever since? I really hoped that it wouldn't have.

'What do you mean by what's normal?' I asked, dragging myself back to the question.

'Let me share something with you,' said Angela getting up and rearranging a photo of what I guessed were her three children on the dresser. Satisfied, she went on, 'We usually think of or define normal as the majority or the consensus, don't we? So let's say that there are twenty people in this room.' She motioned around the room as if to physically count them. 'Ten of them are extremely intelligent and have incredibly high IQs. The other ten have a learning impairment, one outcome of which is that they have a very low IQ. The majority of people outside this room have IQs somewhere in the mid-range so they are the 'norm'.

Would you therefore agree with me that neither group in this room can be defined as 'normal'?'

I agreed, based upon the group she had described.

Angela picked up a ballpoint pen from the small table by the window.

'Let's imagine this is a syringe with a very special drug in it,' she continued as she held it confidently. 'It's full of a drug that is going to cure one of these groups. This injection will make one group normal as per our definition. It will either reduce the IQ of the super intelligent to that of the majority or raise the IQ of those with the learning impairment to that of the majority. The question for you is which should I fix?'

'What a stupid scenario!' I snapped, but Angela pressed me to stick with it as it would challenge a commonly-held assumption. I then asked whether I could give the injection to both groups as I wanted to get clarification to ensure that I did not look silly when I gave my answer.

'No. You have to give the injection to one group only. Which is it going to be?'

Well my first thought was to cure those with the lower IQ to help them to lead a better life and I said so.

'OK,' said Angela. 'Let's change the context a little. Those with the really high IQs develop nuclear weapons and could, if they wanted to, destroy the planet. Those with the really low IQs write lovely poetry. Which will I fix now? Who gets the injection?'

I replied immediately; 'Well given this additional information the higher IQ group naturally because they pose the bigger threat to the rest of us.' The answer seemed obvious even though it differed from my first response.

'So let's revisit the definition of normal,' said Angela as she returned to her seat in front of me. 'One definition of normal, and the one I prefer, is that it is normal to be different. Being different is normal; being unique is normal because human beings are all individual and different. However the problem we face is that our society seems to suggest that there are two types of difference: acceptable and unacceptable. Disability sits within the latter definition. No one wants to be disabled, which seems absolutely reasonable, but those of us who are disabled may feel that this merely adds to our uniqueness and that this difference is entirely acceptable. If your niece had been born with some kind of impairment that would, as you would expect, have caused great anxiety and distress to you and her parents. However the way we would have helped her would have been to understand that she has different skills and abilities which are positive and add to her uniqueness rather than diminishing it.'

It's normal to be different!

Just as I was trying to digest the significance of all of this, Angela changed direction and asked me whether I liked literature. She seemed to have an unerring knack of asking apparently irrelevant questions.

I replied that I did.

'Think of some fictional disabled people in literature or film.'

I scanned my memory of books that I had read and films that I had seen. My first stab at an answer was characters such as Captain Hook and Long John Silver as well as Tiny Tim from Dickens's *A Christmas Carol*. The films that sprang to mind were *The Hunchback of Notre Dame*, *Phantom of the Opera* and *Silence of the Lambs*.

'And what strikes you about these characters?' asked Angela. Before I could reply, she said, 'I will tell you. They are either evil or in need of our pity. That is the way that disability has been portrayed for centuries: something to be feared or something to be pitied. The Hunchback of Notre Dame was ugly and feared to begin with and then at the end we felt sorry for him. No one of course remembers that he was the bell ringer at Notre Dame Cathedral and, as such, performed the valuable function of telling Parisians the time. Have a think about these views of disability before you meet Jan for your next appointment.'

The time had flown by and as I prepared to leave Angela's

house I felt really empowered. I thanked her for her time and hospitality and as I made my way out she said, 'I'm sure, once you've have had the opportunity to meet all of my colleagues and reflect on what they share with you it will all fall into place.' I couldn't wait to continue the conversation, this time with Jan.

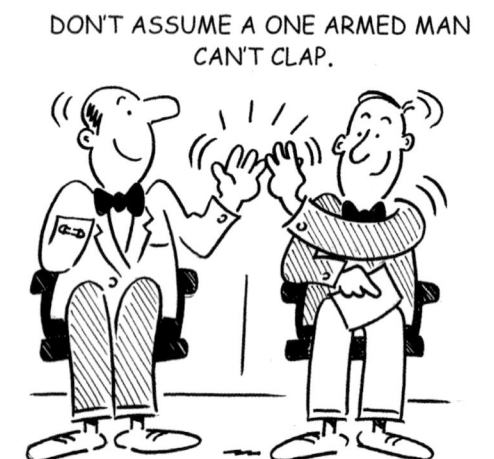

> DON'T ASSUME A ONE ARMED MAN CAN'T CLAP.

I felt extraordinarily elated after that meeting. Suddenly it was ok to be me with what I had. All right, I dearly wanted to be without it but I was no less of a human being because I had it.

After my meeting with Angela I reflected on her views about the history of disability in the human story. I knew from recently talking to a friend, for example, that there was no real reporting of the condition Repetitive Strain Injury when thousands of people, mainly women, were employed in typing pools. In order to stop the keys jamming on the old manual typewriters the keys were arranged so that the typists could not type as quickly and the different pressure required to press the keys on the typewriter meant they used their hands differently. So in essence Repetitive Strain Injury became something of an epidemic in part because of the development of modern computer keyboards.

I also considered the whole concept of 'appropriate sharing' and realised that I had not been talking about my impairment to people in order to protect myself from what might happen. I needed to change my thinking about this too and approach it from the angle that 'this isn't going to hurt me if I tell you and it might actually help'. I also linked it into where I was in George's bereavement process and felt that by sharing it with people – whether at work or with family or friends – was a way of committing myself to the fact that I had what I had. When I am struggling because people don't know about my impairment then things are made worse for me. I can be strong and courageous if that's what I want to be but, by not talking about it at appropriate times, I in fact disable myself.

What was the worst that could happen **if I talked about it?**

What was the worst that could happen **if I didn't?**

By not sharing my impairment appropriately **am I disabling myself?**

If someone has a visible impairment then people remember it most of the time because it is obvious and so it is not really an issue. However, if someone has a non-visible impairment then people can't see it and you may have to keep reminding them of it. Now doing this could be monotonous, but by not doing this we could disable ourselves. I considered that if I was losing my sight maybe I would use a white stick even though I could still see something. At least that way the message was clear and the stick was a communication tool to let others know of my impairment. It was a reasonable adjustment for other people's attitudes rather than one needed for my sight impairment.

After all, it is perfectly normal to be different!

Such a fundamental point made with a few words but it was so difficult to summarise when I met Jan a few days later.

4 Jan

J an lived in a modern bungalow in a quiet part of town. Each building had a small front garden with a driveway leading to the garage. Jan's was no exception although I noticed a shallow ramp leading to the front door. I rang the bell and after a few minutes the door opened to reveal a woman in a wheelchair. I was slightly taken aback but as I collected myself she said, 'You must be Chris. Lovely to meet you, come in.' She expertly manoeuvred the chair and led me through to her spacious lounge. 'Please take a seat and would you like a drink?' Jan asked.

'A cold drink would be lovely,' I replied. 'Would you like a hand?'

Jan smiled and said, 'Not a problem, would orange juice be okay?' I said that would be great and settled back into the armchair. The room was well furnished but I noticed the amount of space between the furniture and realised that everything about the room was done to accommodate a wheelchair. After a short wait Jan returned with our drinks on a lap tray and we began to chat. I told her that I'd really gained a lot from my previous conversations and was grateful for her time. Jan suggested that I summarise what I'd learned.

I began by exploring the idea that there are two perceptions of normal and society had a view on whether that was a positive difference or a negative one. I thought this was very relevant bearing in mind that Jan had a very obvious impairment.

'That is so true,' said Jan enthusiastically. 'When I was a child my parents signed form after form agreeing for me to have operation after operation in order to help me to walk. They understood the fact that I was different from other kids who could get around independently and yet they gave permission for my operations in the hope that I would be cured to make it easier for me to fit in. They were doing what they thought was the best for me – I knew that. They realised that I was going to have a tough life because I was different. It's interesting how people see you if you are different. My impairment is seen as a negative difference whereas something like pregnancy, which can also be disabling for some people, is understandably viewed as a positive difference.'

As if as an afterthought she added, 'Sorry I didn't mean to give you a lecture! I just feel so passionately about this idea that everybody is different. But so what? Because I have an impairment, and a visible one at that, I am disabled by other people's attitudes towards me and what they think I am able to do.'

Even though I was somewhat taken aback, I was keen to hear her perspective – whatever that was.

'Carry on,' I said. 'This is fascinating. I've been thinking about the fact that I'm in the same club as evil characters such as Captain Hook and Long John Silver or needy characters like Tiny Tim. I understand the whole issue of what society defines as normal and the fact that people who have an impairment are often mistakenly seen as not normal. There are some common themes where disabled people are stereotyped. The role models that we have in the main are negative. They're either villains or heroic or pitiful. An alternative is that we are extraordinary, blessed with enhanced senses or great courage.'

'Precisely,' added Jan. 'A friend of mine has a mental health condition and because of that some people treat him as if he's Hannibal Lector! Now I have a sense of humour as good as anyone's and yet stereotyping my friend in this way is not funny – it is incredibly disabling. Now let me ask you how would you describe people with a disability? How do you think of yourself and your impairment?'

I was a little confused by the question and the sheer speed of Jan's conversation. She had so much she wanted to say and it felt like she was trying to give me everything she knew all at once. After a few moments' reflection, I said that I primarily saw myself as having an illness and that I would like to be cured.

'So how does that link with a positive view of being disabled?' asked Jan.

Thinking through what Jan had just said, I could see that wanting to get rid of something wasn't a very positive view of it at all.

'You've just described something that many have termed

the medical model,' said Jan. 'This model – or perspective if you like – is one which positions disabled people as ill or sick and in need of curing. The question here is 'Can it be fixed?' and, 'If we can't fix or cure it, can we sort out the symptoms?' It's about the things I can't do now that I have this condition and often this whole area is never discussed in layman's terms. It's all wrapped up in medical jargon. It's all about medical professionals giving us advice in order to avoid the risks. Society sets great store by the opinions of the medical fraternity and it can be extremely difficult for an individual to challenge them. So knowing this model is focused on illness and cure, how do you feel as you join our disability club?'

'Well as I said, the first thing I want to know is whether I can be fixed, whether I can be cured.'

'Yes. That's absolutely it,' said Jan excitedly. 'Disability is seen as bad news. Society puts us in a box labelled 'damaged goods'. Like you, I guess I didn't ask to have what I have. But the thing is that I've got it and that can't really be changed however much I vote against it. I could spend my time wishing for the past when I wasn't disabled, hoping my doctor finds a cure or if they don't I'll rely on my faith to help me recover. Now let me say, I am a very religious person and proud of it. I once took a trip to a place where miracles are supposed to happen. I came home a few days later still with my impairment but also with a nasty dose of the flu! I discussed the lack of a cure with a local priest and he suggested that the problem was my faith wasn't strong enough! It seems you can't win. And of course it's always your problem.'

Jan went on to talk about the fact that disabled people are very much under the control of doctors. If a doctor says no to you working then you can't work. Try getting insurance if a doctor says your condition puts you at risk.

'But I see my doctor as one of my most important advisers, my greatest ally. If I did not have their support what sort of mess would I be in?'

I was actually quite appalled at Jan's attack on doctors. I reasoned that without the support of the medical profession I didn't believe that people with impairments would lead such long and often pain-free lives.

'Don't get me wrong', Jan continued emphatically. 'I am not saying that medical professionals are not good. Of course they are. They play an absolutely pivotal role in society and contribute in ways that the rest of us never do. We just need to understand one additional thing with the whole medical agenda – what is the impact on us if people approach disability solely from the medical angle?'

This question again challenged something in me. 'So what you're saying is that if all you have is the medical model or medical perspective as a point of reference then many will only see us as ill or needing to be cured or fixed?'

If we only use the **medical model**, people with impairments are seen primarily as ill and need curing.

That is disabling!

'You've got it,' stated Jan. 'And it's really hard to get work if you're not fit. I'm not suggesting that if science came up with a cure for a particular impairment that it wouldn't be good news; of course it would. It's just that it's interesting to consider how those who are non-disabled view people with an impairment – if they see us as 'ill' first and foremost. It's not all right to be disabled so therefore we need to cure it and, on one level, many would agree with that, but it suggests that 'I am the problem and I must be fixed'.

I remembered that Angela had talked about mankind's history being full of examples of disability and how nature had normally dealt with it. Jan agreed and said that medical advancement meant that many more severely impaired people were surviving. This places even greater demands on our society to develop all manner of services which can support those with the most complex needs.

Jan leant forward in her chair as if to emphasise her next point. 'In some parts of the world we are able to screen for a disability before a child is born. If the test proves positive we can make a decision on whether it should be born or not. What I'd like to know is what is so wrong with having people around who are different? The only way we're going to survive is by being different. Do you know why the potato famine happened in Ireland all those years ago?' she asked.

I said that I didn't, but I knew that approximately a million people had died.

'Well,' continued Jan, 'the potato at the time was developed from one particular type and it couldn't resist the disease known as potato blight. The crop failed and the rest is history. Potatoes that were different would probably have survived. People coping with impairments still have talents which we need to use for the good of everyone.' Jan sat back and took a breath. Then she asked, 'What other perspectives are there on disabled people?'

Other words that described the illness perspective raced through my mind: sick, hospital, tests, diagnosis, rehabilitation. All the words were connected with the medical model. Then I remembered Tiny Tim and how the Hunchback of Notre Dame was eventually depicted.

'What about those who need our help?' I asked. 'People like Tiny Tim.'

Jan agreed and asked me how I would describe him. I said

he was ill so that was the medical model but really I felt sorry for him and I wanted to help him. That was what got to Scrooge in the end – the sadness of the situation.

Jan pressed me as to what I would do if I felt sorry for him. I replied that I would want to help him somehow.

She asked me how.

I searched for an answer. I recounted that I had helped old ladies across the road and completed sponsored walks for charity. I concluded that I often help by giving my time or money.

Jan smiled at my response and went on to describe something she called the charity model. It focused on people feeling better about themselves by helping other people who they perceive as being less fortunate.

I was confused and a little annoyed. 'But surely that money goes to good causes? It's put to good use. It helps fund research and makes a difference to many people's lives. Surely you're not suggesting that charity is bad?' I was beginning to wonder whether this conversation was going to be as stimulating as the previous three.

'Not at all,' replied Jan emphatically. 'Where would research be without donations? How would good work be done here and abroad if money had not been raised and given by individuals, companies and governments? My point is more about how the money is raised. If I show a picture of someone who is disabled, I need to show him or her looking pitiful – as if they need help. The appeal needs to forcefully make the point that without charity these people's lives would be wretched. When do you see pictures of successful people that have impairments featuring in charity campaigns?'

'Not very often at all now you come to mention it. Maybe Stephen Hawking but I can't think of any others.'

'Good example and yet I can't think of others either. That's because successful disabled people aren't pitiful enough for you to give money to them. Look I am in a wheelchair. I have a great job. I have a good enough income. I am what I would term happy. Do you think you'd see me being used in a charity appeal to encourage people to donate? Well I know that I wouldn't donate as much if I saw someone like me. In fact I'm unlikely to donate at all because it looks like the individual is enjoying life and doesn't need my support.'

Jan changed tack. 'When you look at the charity would you describe it as a charity 'for' disabled people or 'of' disabled people? Let me explain,' she continued. 'If it's an organisation 'for' disabled people, then it's very likely that non-disabled people make the decisions as to what disabled people need. If it's an organisation 'of' disabled people then disabled people run it and decide what assistance is needed. Just like one of our most popular slogans says "Nothing about us without us!" Put another way,' said Jan, 'you would expect the chair of a charity for women to be a woman. Surely it's the same for disabled people? And at the end of the day I really want the person who speaks on my behalf to have some personal experience of the difficulties I might face.'

I was really intrigued by this approach and eager to make sense of what Jan had said. I now understood that the charity model was often about portraying disabled people as suffering and as victims. This approach appeared designed to invoke feelings of pity and the result was people donate more. Disabled people are seen as helpless, less fortunate and dependent on the support and charity of others. We are brave, plucky characters who, despite our impairments, soldier on and manage to be happy and achieve in spite of everything. And of course the contract is that others give and we are really grateful. The emphasis is once again on the 'dis' part of disability and focuses on everything that disabled people can't do when compared to those who don't have impairments.

I slowly nodded and smiled at Jan as we both realised that I had got the message.

If we only use the **charity model**, people with impairments are primarily seen as less fortunate and need our pity and help.

That is disabling!

Jan went on to suggest that there is real tension related to this model because of the genuine desire of human beings to be kind and supportive; when disabled people challenge this thinking, they can be seen as ungrateful or as having a chip on their shoulder.

'I call it the oppression of kindness,' she said. 'And the conflict is about how we can be independent if we are supposed to be needy and grateful.'

Jan let this point hang in the air. Then she pressed on.

'The oppression of kindness is everywhere in the world of disabled people. Let me give you an example' Jan said. 'When I was very small, and also disabled so I couldn't walk, my mum stopped me from climbing a tree in our back garden. She was obviously very worried about the risk that I might fall and seriously hurt myself. She didn't stop my younger non-disabled brother from climbing the same tree though. This simple act of a caring mother placed limits on my behaviour based mainly on my disability and, of course, an unintended consequence was that she stopped me from seeing the world from up there. All of these actions were limiting and were driven by kindness with the outcome often being that my horizons were severely restricted. We are subtly discriminated against by kindness which, although a terrific human attribute, doesn't always help. Society continually makes judgements about what is best for us, some of which are helpful but some of which are definitely not. I should be able to decide what support I need. Well-meaning people do things to us or for us, rather than seeking to work in partnership and collaboration with us.'

Jan went on to explain that what we want is not only a better understanding of the support we really need but also to be fully engaged in the decision-making processes whose outcomes benefit disabled and non-disabled people alike. That is what we see happening with regard to the other equality strands such as race, gender and sexual orientation.

This whole conversation was summarised with one powerful question:

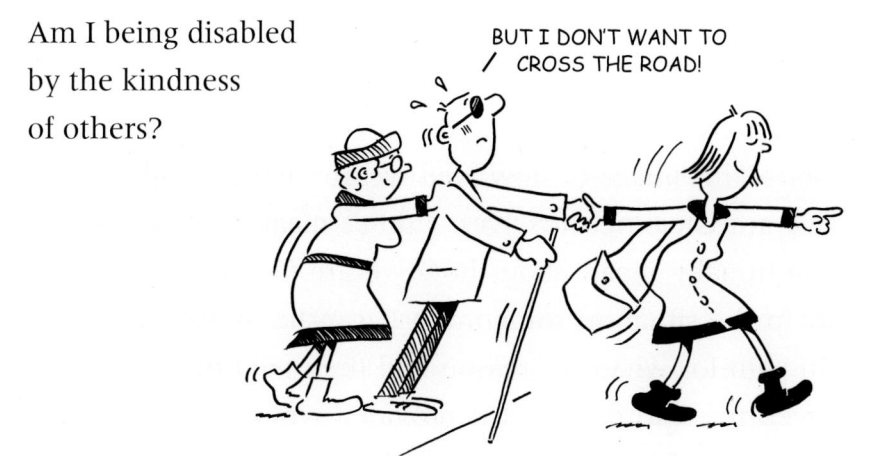

Am I being disabled by the kindness of others?

AM I BEING DISABLED BY THE KINDNESS OF OTHERS?

I thought about the question and reflected on the fact that it was difficult enough for people to take a stand against racial hatred or homophobic behaviour or the bigot where it was clear that intense dislike or hatred were the drivers. It seemed somehow more difficult to develop responses to oppression where the drivers were kindness and concern.

'Have you ever smiled for other people when you don't feel like smiling for yourself?' Jan continued.

'All the time,' I replied resignedly.

Jan nodded. 'I thought so. A bit like the tears of a clown, don't you think? Who's the smile for? If it's for us because we are happy then fine. But how many disabled people do you think are smiling only because they want to fit in and act as if they are this brave person soldiering on despite what's really going on for them? We are so keen to show this image of how well we are doing to others that we are cheating ourselves. I don't mean that we should continually moan about how we are feeling but it might help the situation sometimes. It can be ok to say we are in pain for whatever reason and then tell others what we need them to do about it provided we don't always play this card. Smiling about it and looking brave just takes energy that we could put to better use in order to deal with the pain. We're doing it for others not for ourselves.'

> When I am smiling, **who am I smiling for?** Myself or others?

Jan paused for breath and then summarised the conversation so far. The frames of reference that we have when we enter the world of disability are the charity and medical models. Both models have their place and position the world of disability in different ways. But they both have one thing in common: they portray the disabled person as the problem. Jan then became even more animated as she started to take me through a third model which she called the social model.

'I've never heard of that,' I said truthfully. 'What's it all about?'

'Well you may have noticed that I am a woman,' Jan continued chuckling. 'Do you think that I have ever experienced any form of discrimination because I am a woman?'

I replied that I was sure she had at some time in her life.

'Well I actually have the answer to stop all that gender-based discrimination,' she continued. Then, as if she was delivering the punch line to a joke, she said, 'What I need to do is to become a man!'

'What?' I exclaimed. 'But that's a stupid idea!'

'I know that and you know that. But it would stop the discrimination don't you think?'

I had to agree but showed my opposition to the suggestion.

'Don't worry,' she giggled. 'The point I am making is that the problem is not that I am a woman; the problem is some men's viewpoint on women. It's like suggesting that someone who is black and from an ethnic minority background should become white in order to stop the racial discrimination they may experience. We need to 'cure' the sexist, the bigot and the racist, not the target of their attacks. The same is true of disability; fix the negative attitudes towards disability and then we won't be treated as second class citizens or feel the need to go off and get 'cured'. I've had fourteen operations to help me to walk partly because society is inconvenienced by wheelchair users and because it expects me to walk just to fit in.'

My head was starting to spin. On the one hand what Jan was saying was making such perfect sense, but on the other it was a fundamental shift in the way I thought – the way I had been brought up to think.

She went on to explain that the social model was an approach developed by disabled people themselves and focused on how we want things organised or how others should treat us. It began first in America when thousands of young people went to Vietnam to fight for their country and large numbers of them returned with terrible injuries, both physical and mental. They became increasingly angry, because on the one hand they were being seen as heroes but on the other they experienced disability-based discrimination. They were heroes who couldn't get on their local bus or visit their local cinema because it wasn't wheelchair accessible!

Jan then changed tack yet again and asked me, 'How tall are you?'

'Five foot seven,' I replied.

'Imagine that you lived in a world populated exclusively by people like me who are in wheelchairs. How would we change the light bulbs in this room?' She gestured towards the ceiling.

Each of my replies to this strange question brought a grin and a firm 'no' from Jan. She asked me why we needed tools that could be extended so as to reach the light bulbs? Why would we have lights on the walls instead of the ceilings? Noticing that I was becoming increasingly frustrated with the conversation, she proclaimed, 'Why not just have lower ceilings?'

'But then I would have to bend down every time I came into the room.'

'Ah so now you don't fit! You don't fit – not just this room but every room of every building on our planet! You don't fit any more. You're not normal!'

I started to feel uncomfortable at this prospect despite the fact that it was all hypothetical.

Jan continued the metaphor with a broad smile and at her usual fast pace.

'That's why we have built this building for you and we call it the Centre for the Tall. This residential unit is where you all live. Everything is designed to accommodate your height problem. Now don't get me wrong, I personally like tall people. I have been on a tall-awareness training course so I understand what it's like to be tall. I get your language too, phrases like 'walking tall', 'put your best foot forward' and 'stand up and be counted'. They don't really mean much to us in wheelchairs because we say things like 'we're rushed off our wheels' but at least I'm happy for you to have your own sayings. I've also done 'tall-a-thons' to raise money for the Centre so that it stays open and has lots of decent facilities. We provide you with benefits and of course a shoe allowance. I buy your hand-made mats and baskets when you hold your fund-raising fêtes. Before I went on the course I thought tall people weren't very bright because the air was thinner up there! I realise now it might have to do with the fact that because you can't get in our schools you've had a very limited education. I would really like to help you though so what would you like me to do?'

Jan was obviously enjoying the absurdity of the scenario and she was laughing as she added each one of her ideas. I, on the other hand, began to feel increasingly irritated. This was preposterous. How could she treat and speak to me this way when there was nothing wrong with me? As I reflected on this I started to get angry especially as Jan was reluctant to let the scenario drop.

'You could give me a wheelchair,' I shouted defiantly. 'Then I could get into your stupid buildings!'

'Ah, so that's the adjustment that you want me to make is it?' mocked Jan. 'You getting a wheelchair means that you can now come and visit and work in our buildings. I don't know if that really is the solution because you'll only keep forgetting you're a wheelchair user won't you? You'll get up out of your wheelchair and bang your head and we wouldn't want that would we? I could restrain you I guess. That would stop you hurting yourself. Perhaps a better solution would be a height reduction operation. Maybe we should amputate your legs! You'd certainly be able to get in to the building then!'

Jan then took a more serious tone, 'You do know that we've developed a test to screen all babies for 'tallness' so there is no need for any more to be born. Tallness is grounds for termination of pregnancy. You are part of the last generation of tall people there will ever be because we have cured tallness.'

I was getting genuinely angry now and could sense a growing tension between us. Jan was treating me as if I was the problem. She was discriminating against me and I felt devalued and persecuted. I practically yelled that I wanted to be given a wheelchair.

'OK,' conceded Jan. 'Here's your wheelchair. Your problem has just been solved.'

At last, a result! I felt relieved and bit less angry and thought I'd out-manoeuvred her in this absurd scenario that had generated real feelings of anger in me.

So why was she still smiling?

'You can get into our buildings now but your troubles have only just begun,' she smirked, 'haven't they ... lanky?'

'What do you mean?' I retorted hesitantly.

'You're no longer disabled by the fact that the ceilings are too low. You're now disabled by the attitudes of those of us who have always used wheelchairs. You're being discriminated against because you are different and not accepted for who you are. Tall people are seen as bad news. They should be in institutions. Are you and the other tall people looking to take our jobs? Is tallness contagious? We don't want tall people living in our street. I certainly don't want my daughter going out with one!'

That was it! There was no way that she was going to make me feel like this. I could barely control my anger so I stood up, threw down my pen and pad and got ready to leave the house. 'This is totally ridiculous,' I said.

'Is it?' Jan replied, 'Come and sit down and let's explore what's really getting up your nose.'

I took a deep breath and reluctantly sat down. I explained in no uncertain terms just how angry her scenario had made me. She responded by saying that my anger was perfectly understandable. She then asked me whether this was any different to the anger I sometimes felt when others were discriminating against me as a result of my own impairment. I said I did get upset and angry sometimes and I, slowly but surely, began to make the connection between the scenario and my real situation.

I hadn't wanted to be fixed in her scenario even though Jan had been trying to help my situation with these suggestions. She was representing the medical model which sees the disabled person as the problem and therefore in need of a cure.

Having said that, it is clear there is a role for medical intervention but it must be in line with the individual's wishes. Actually the real cure in this scenario was to raise the ceilings not amputate my legs!

The charity model was also present in the role play. Jan had talked about doing all those charitable things for me as if I was powerless to help myself. She might feel better because of the help she and society were providing but at the end of the day it didn't really tackle the situation. I wanted to be independent and live a life like other people.

The social model was the one I wanted. This model didn't see me as the problem; it saw the ceilings and the attitudes of others as the problem. They needed fixing, not me! By raising the ceilings and changing the attitudes of others I could be accepted for who I was and not be discriminated against because of my 'tallness'.

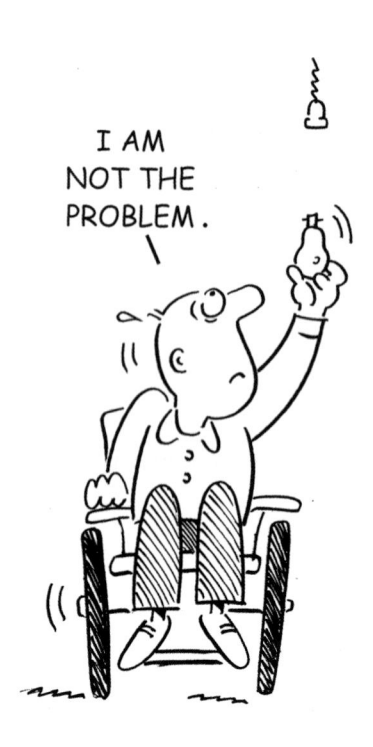

Jan summarised it very well over a cup of coffee at the end of our meeting when she said, 'I need to change me, change others and the physical barriers – not my legs.'

We parted as friends even though my time with Jan had been frustrating, even irritating at times and certainly full of emotion. But the lessons she taught, I could see, would be invaluable as I made sense of my impairment and the world's reaction to it.

Fix the physical barriers, deal with the attitudes of people out there and it's sorted.

I am not the problem.

That is empowering!

Later that evening I sat at home still reflecting on the conversation with Jan and thinking over its implications.

If the world 'lived' by the social model, people with impairments would not be disabled in the way they are now. Society has, instead, put care above education and charity above inclusion. Jan had said that everyone assumed she would be better off if she was not disabled and yet she earned a good salary, drove a car and loved her family. What was so wrong with that? The social model was about managing other people's attitudes and was just as liberating as similar changes in viewpoints on the issues of race and gender.

My concentration was broken when I heard the baby from next door crying. I found myself thinking about how a wheelchair-using mother would lift the baby from the cot in order to comfort him or her. The design of the cot would help or hinder the processes. I heard a bus travelling in the street outside my house and thought that if I couldn't get onto a bus in a wheelchair because of the lack of a ramp then it was the bus that was the problem not me. No wonder Jan felt so relaxed about her impairment when she was thinking in that way.

Ok, there were flaws with some aspects of the social model; blind people can't see the sunrise or beautiful paintings and wheelchair users most certainly won't climb every mountain or flight of stairs. Deaf people won't hear birdsong or music. But access or inclusion is not just about doors and steps – it is also about attitudes. The social model does deal with this. It doesn't 'fix' the middle-aged person with depression or the ten year old with autism, but it does focus on the disablist attitudes of others as being part of the problem.

I had sometimes felt that the cure for what I have would have been not being born in the first place. I then reminded myself of the contribution I had made even though it had not been earth-shattering: I had made some difference to those I loved and who loved me. No, the real issue here was understanding that part of the solution is changing other people's view of me when they know I have an impairment.

That meant I had to stop apologising for the impact of my impairment and start taking control. I could then be more of an ambassador for all those people with impairments who come after me.

I looked forward to my final conversation, this time with Paul.

5 Paul

Paul's office was a little way out of town and located in an old building along with a number of other organisations. It had a small car park at the front with a short flight of steps and a ramp leading up to the main entrance. Once inside I was directed to a ground floor office where a short man with glasses, dressed in jeans and a checked shirt introduced himself as Paul and welcomed me in.

After we had exchanged small talk and made a start on the tea and biscuits, Paul asked how I was feeling about the conversations I'd had so far.

I replied that I had learned more in the last ten days about the world of disability than I had learnt in the rest of my life even though I was now a fully paid up member of the Disability Club. I had also learnt a great deal about myself and my partner had noticed a change in me too – a really positive change.

'I know just what you mean,' replied Paul. 'It's all about your mind-set and about how you view yourself and your life. There are different types of mind-set: for example, imagine a young child who gets a present for their birthday and all they want to do is to play with the box. What's the box?'

'Oh it's anything they want it to be,' I said remembering my own childhood and the excitement of imaginative play. 'A plane, a castle, a ship, a spaceship,' I continued enthusiastically.

'Oh yes, good one! So if it's a spaceship, who is everybody else in the room?'

'Aliens!'

'Fantastic,' said Paul eagerly. 'Very magical wouldn't you say, as an approach to life? A box can be a spaceship and parents can be aliens just like that. Anything is possible and anyone can be anything.'

'They don't call Disneyland the Magical Kingdom for no reason,' I suggested. 'Anything is possible there and anyone can enjoy it.'

'Exactly,' agreed Paul. 'Now imagine a somewhat older child of say eight, nine or ten. Who do they imagine themselves to be when they play?'

'Oh sports stars, film stars or pop stars these days – those sort of celebrities.'

'Yes. It's all about heroes. They see themselves winning the Cup Final or the World Cup or perhaps an Oscar. In this mind-set most things are possible and most people can do what they want. When I score a goal in a football game in the park I imagine hearing the roar of the Wembley crowd in my ears as I do it. Other youngsters might stand in front of the bedroom mirror and mime to the songs of their favourite pop stars and pretend they are actually on stage with them. It's a heroic mind-set. Not the same as the magical one though as I've sort of worked out that I'm not Peter Pan. I tried flying by leaping off the garden wall and I've still got the bruises to prove that it didn't work out!'

Paul was having fun, warming to the task and clearly

enjoying the conversation. I was enjoying it too and said so.

Paul continued. 'Imagine you're older now and in your first job and you want to make a real difference. You come up with what you think is a great idea but your boss says that you have to fill in a form in triplicate and then wait for days for what is usually a negative reply. You come to understand that, 'Sometimes it can be done and usually it's the same people who can do it'. You become resigned to the fact that this is the way it's done around here and you can't really change it.'

'Oh I remember that only too well,' I replied as images of frustration came flooding back based on too many memories of that type of experience.

'And then of course,' said Paul, 'there is the last mind-set. Using our age metaphor we see a person who has retired and who has come to believe that 'nothing is possible and nobody can do it'. Very cynical, wouldn't you say?'

I sighed heavily at the very thought of dealing with people like this.

Paul continued, 'One definition of a cynic I really like is, 'A cynic is someone who has closed their mind but not their mouth'. You can hear them saying, 'We tried that thirty years ago and it didn't work then so there's no way it's going to work now.'

'Oh I've met my fair share of those,' I replied. 'It would have been nice to have avoided experiences and people like that. I've always found them a little frustrating.'

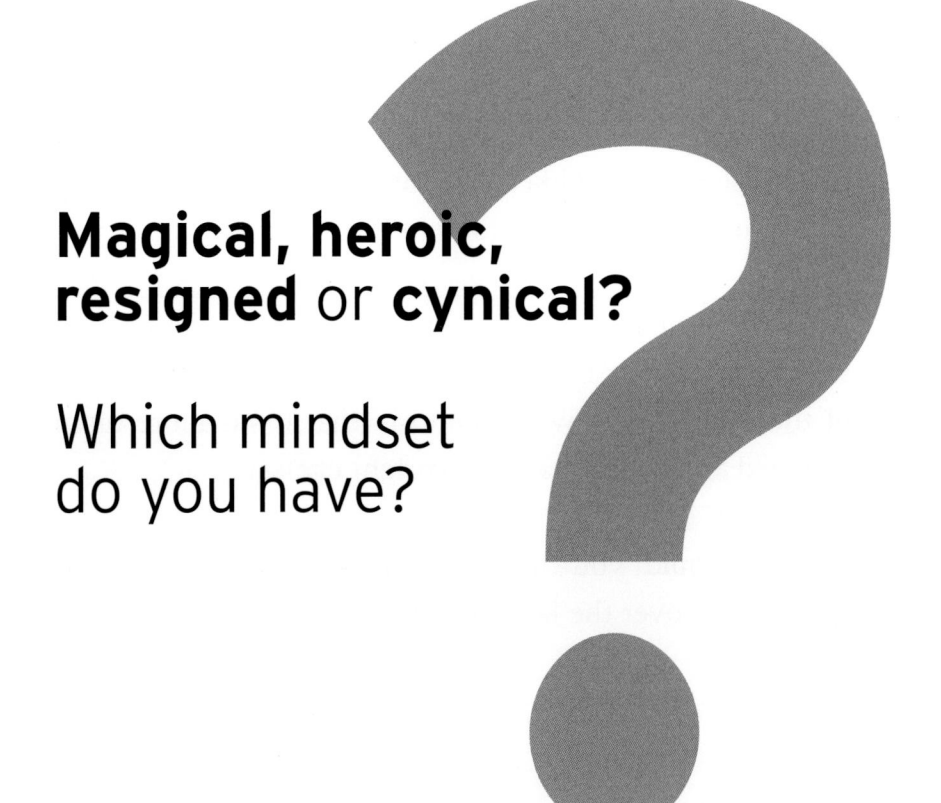

Magical, heroic, resigned or cynical?

Which mindset do you have?

'So there you are,' Paul said. 'Four different mind-sets. And do you think age really dictates which mind-set you choose?'

'Absolutely not,' I replied. 'I've met some very magical older people and some very cynical youngsters.'

'I totally agree. So in which mind-set do you think you spend most of your time?'

Silence can feel pretty awkward, especially when you are the one who has to break it. I stirred my tea and munched on another biscuit, playing for time. The reason you hesitate is because you don't like the answer you know you should give in order to reply honestly to the question.

Before I became disabled I honestly believe I would have said heroic. I felt my imaginary glass was half full most of the time. But now I would say that I was more often resigned and occasionally downright cynical.

'Where would your partner put you now after your experiences over the last ten days?' asked Paul.

'Kind of back to heroic I would say. We both know that

there are things that I just can't do anymore but at least I don't keep moaning about it all the time. I don't see the 'dis' now and focus more on the 'ability'. My partner says that I'm also more fun to be around now.'

Paul got up and moved around the room, adjusted his glasses and then, looking at me, continued, 'It's important to live one of the first two mind-sets otherwise you're always limiting yourself and also you're no fun to be around. To be honest, I've also known people who exist in the last two mind-sets and their symptoms seem to get worse more quickly. Your body does seem to listen to your inner conversations. I know it's so easy to slip into the resigned and cynical mind-sets, especially if, like most people, you become disabled during your adult life. It's understandable that people tend to focus on what they can't do rather than what they can: 'I used to be able to do this but now I can't'. That's why they end up in a rut and forget to keep living.'

I wanted to say something but could not find the words. Paul sensed this and continued to drive home his point.

'You've got to have the right mind-set if you're going to apply what you have learnt over the past fortnight. The reason you're seeing me after George, Angela and Jan is because you have to understand what they've learnt before you can apply their principles. Applying them is where I come in. It starts with having a positive, magical and heroic mind-set and that is down to you.'

'That's really interesting,' I said. 'I'd like to be able to apply my knowledge as well as I could. Would you mind helping me with that?'

'Of course not,' said Paul stretching his legs, 'Let's try this. What's two plus two?'

'Pardon? Is this a trick question?' I asked, a little baffled.

'What's two plus two?' repeated Paul smiling.

'Four,' I replied, still rather confused.

Paul continued asking exactly the same question over and over again. I always gave the same answer 'Four'.

After the ninth question I started to show my frustration with the game.

Suddenly Paul changed the question.

'What's three plus two?'

At last! 'Five,' I proclaimed.

'Exactly! A different result. A different outcome. So let's take a moment to explore this,' said Paul. 'If the first 'two' of our sum represents what you do or say and the second 'two' represents what they do or say, you always get the same result: four. But if you change your 'two' to a 'three', you will get a different result – five. The moment you do or say something different and they do or say the same back you will still get a different result. In fact, if they want the same result as before they have to change what they are doing. For example, you change to a 'three', they need to change to a 'one' in order to get the same answer as before – 'four'.'

It made perfect sense. If you want a different result to your situation you have to do something different yourself. If you wait for the other person to change you could wait forever. If you keep doing what you've always done you'll always get the same result.

Moving on Paul asked, 'Tell me what you learnt from George.'

I remembered all the intriguing things about language that he had made me aware of and I shared some of the examples with Paul that I had noticed since my discussions with George.

'Excellent. You've really noticed the impact that words can have but that is only a third of the story. You've also got to think about the way you say things: not only the words but also the music and the dance.'

'Words, music and dance?' I enquired hesitantly.

Paul made himself more comfortable and went on to explain what each of these elements meant.

Words are simply the words that I choose to use – what I actually say. These are obviously important in communicating any message. The thing is it isn't just the words you use but how many words you use. Some people say things in twenty sentences when two would have been enough. In fact, saying it in twenty sentences actually confuses the message. With language, less is more.

Paul suggested that I should also make sure that I use positive phrases rather than negative ones. To illustrate his point Paul said, 'Don't think of a pink elephant,' and what did I do? You've got it – I thought of a pink elephant even though he had told me not to. I was getting the point. What he should have done was to tell me what he wanted me to think about rather than what he didn't. He should have said, 'Think of a blue giraffe.'

I found this fascinating especially as I remember a time when my niece was visiting and while helping to lay the table my sister said to her, 'Don't drop that plate.' What did she do? Well, she dropped it. My sister should have said, 'Hold that plate tightly!' It's a much clearer message especially because we interpret negative messages in a different order. 'Don't drop that plate' is actually interpreted as 'Drop that plate – Don't'! I have to first imagine myself dropping the plate before I imagine myself not dropping it.

Paul described his final point about diluting words and diluting phrases. He quoted specific examples that I realised I'd used in my meeting with him and they had all had the effect of diluting the impact I made. These were phrases like:

'It would have been nice to have avoided experiences and people like that.'
'I've always found them a little frustrating.'

'I'd like to be able to apply my knowledge as well as I could. Would you mind helping me with that?'

'Do you see how diluting those phrases are?' asked Paul after he had quoted my words back to me. 'What is the likelihood of someone doing what you need them to do if you say 'would you mind'? Now don't get me wrong they might do it but the emphasis is not there is it?'

I had to admit he was right. 'What should I have said in order to increase my impact then?' I enquired.

Paul thought for a moment and then said: 'You could have used words like,

'I needed to avoid experiences and people like that.'
'I've always found them very frustrating.'
'I really want to be able to apply my knowledge as well as I can.'
'What I need you to do is to help me with that.'

'What has this got to do with disability?' I wondered, until Paul provided lots of examples of what he had heard people with impairments say in relation to their disability:

'It would be nice if you could sort out a chair for me.'
'I'd really appreciate it if you could look at me when you are speaking.'
'I'd be grateful if you could sort that for me.'
'It would be good to get that done by the weekend if that's ok with you?'
'I'm getting by at the moment thanks.'
'I could do with being a bit closer if you don't mind.'

Compare the dilution of these phrases to:
'I need that chair to be sorted out.'
'I need you to look at me when you are speaking.'
'I do need you to sort that out for me.'
'I need that done by the weekend, please.'
'I need some support with this particular area please.'
'I need to be closer, please.'

I protested that while I wanted people to get my message, I did not want to appear rude. Surely that would reduce my chances of people helping me when I needed it?

'I know what you are saying,' agreed Paul. 'My parents used to say to me that 'he who wants doesn't get'. The trouble is that if I don't say what I want or need, I'm even less likely to get it.'

My choice of **WORDS** is important:

How many do I use? Do I use **too many** words?

Do I use **positive** commands rather than negative ones?

Do I reduce the impact of my messages with **diluting words and phrases**?

He went on to ask me whether people were psychic enough to understand what I needed when I did not help them with the language I used. Also asking for what I needed did not mean I could not also say 'please'. I could see that the words we use were obviously vital.

I had always thought of myself as an assertive person but I was beginning to recognise that none of the assertiveness courses I'd ever attended had helped me to deal assertively with my disability.

Next Paul described the 'music', which is the way that we say the words. This includes such elements as the tone of voice, the speed of the voice, the volume, the emphasis on certain words and the passion and energy behind the voice. Paul modelled this by using the following phrase and contrasted the different meanings of the seven phrases just by moving the emphasis:

'*I* didn't say you stole that money.' (It wasn't me. It must have been someone else who said it.)

'I *didn't* say you stole that money.' (I am denying that I said that particular message.)

'I didn't *say* you stole that money.' (I could have written it down or implied it but I didn't actually say it.)

'I didn't say *you* stole that money.' (It wasn't you but someone else who stole it.)

'I didn't say you *stole* that money.' (You could have borrowed it.)

'I didn't say you stole *that* money.' (You stole some other money!)

'I didn't say you stole that *money*.' (You stole something else but not the money.)

Use the same seven words but change the emphasis and you get seven different meanings or messages. No wonder the written word and emails cause misunderstandings and are so often misconstrued.

When it comes to disability, it is pointless using assertive words to ask somebody to do something if you use a weak sounding tone or an apologetic voice. The same message has to come through in both the words and the music. Before moving on Paul said, 'Dealing with words and music isn't always easy or possible for some people who have certain impairments which affect their communication skills. For example, for someone who is deaf and uses sign language it will clearly have a major impact on a conversation with a hearing person. In order to get round this potential difficulty the deaf person should explain how they intend to communicate so that the hearing person understands the rules.' Paul continued, 'By taking control in this way the deaf person is also coming over as assertive which is really helpful.'

'Someone who has, for instance, cerebral palsy and has difficulty speaking stands a good chance of being misunderstood and the music they use may have a negative impact on people listening. Once again dealing with this at the beginning of any important conversation is crucial. Telling the listener about the impact of their condition on speech will not only reassure but also demonstrate assertiveness.'

My use of **MUSIC** is important:

Do I use appropriate **speed and volume** in my voice?

Should I increase the **passion and energy** in my voice to convey that I mean what I say?

How can I emphasise the **key words** to help the clarity of my message?

How can I **explain my rules** if my impairment impacts on the conversation?

'So,' Paul said, 'let's now look at the final element often called body language and which I call 'dance'. This includes all the visual factors such as a person's posture, their gestures, their facial expressions and whether they are making appropriate eye contact.'

Paul then demonstrated physical movements that had very differing effects on me; during the first one I could tell he was embarrassed about what he was saying; the next one he looked obviously confident; in the third he was nervous and in the fourth, he was aggressive. All of this happened purely because he changed his body language, his 'dance'.

Once again Paul acknowledged that, for some people their impairment dramatically affects their dance or body language. He said, 'Someone sitting in a wheelchair as a result of multiple sclerosis may not have the ability to move in different ways. The important thing is to let the listener know how important the subject is by emphasising the words. They could say, for example, "Although my tone of voice or movements might make it look as if this doesn't matter to me, I need you to understand that it really does matter."'

I really got the point: communication matters hugely and

thinking about what we're going to say as well as how we're going to say it will improve our chances of actually being listened to and of our message being really heard!

My use of **DANCE** is important:

How do I use visual clues such as **gestures and posture** to enhance my message?

Do I retain appropriate **eye contact** throughout?

How do I use appropriate **facial expressions** to reinforce my message?

'At the end of the day,' continued Paul, 'what we need is for all three of these elements to work together. If I say I need you to review my reasonable adjustments for my disability, these are the words I need to use. I also need to say it with a confident, energetic tone and pace (music) and confident gestures and facial expressions (dance) that also confirm this is what I need you to do. So often we are let down by one or more of these three elements and people therefore get mixed messages. No wonder we don't get what we need to address our disability if we don't use the right means of communication.'

I could see the obvious usage of these techniques but wanted to make sure my point about rudeness was really clarified.

'But, like I said earlier, won't it come across as a little rude if I go around saying what I need all the time?' I enquired.

'Do you mean 'a little rude' or do you mean 'rude'?' pressed Paul. 'You are diluting your meaning again, Chris.'

'I mean rude!' I exclaimed. I was disappointed with myself. What Paul was helping me with was absolute common sense but it would take a lot more to make it common practice for me.

'Okay, let's pick up the issue of whether you're being rude,' said Paul. 'I'm going to share ten words with you that when used will help you to deal with any situation you find yourself in and if used properly removes rudeness from the equation. These ten words will help you to tackle situations where previously you might have avoided them; and used with the appropriate music and dance they are incredibly powerful. The ten words are:

What I like…
What I don't like…
What I need…

Firstly 'What I like' is positive and could include:
▶▶   what I like about what the other person has done
▶▶   what I appreciate about their agenda
▶▶   what I've valued about something they have done in the past.
In fact I can add anything that shows I appreciate, value or understand the other person's/ people's agenda.

'What I don't' like is about:
▶▶   what is not happening as I would want
▶▶   what I am frustrated/ disappointed about
▶▶   the issues I am facing with my agenda.

In fact I can add anything that is not as I would want it.

'What I need' focuses on:
▶▶ What I need to happen to rectify the 'what I don't like' situation. This could be what I need or in fact what I want or even what I insist on if the situation demands that strength of language'.

Paul explained that each time you use this structure you can vary the words (as long as you keep 'need' or 'want' in the final stage). The structures help avoid using the diluting words/ phrases that he reminded me of earlier. You would also need to ensure the music and dance is as upbeat as possible and matches the assertiveness of the words.

He went on to talk through some examples of what he had either personally used or heard other people say:

'I really do appreciate the effort you have put in to try to rectify the situation with the equipment that I need. Having said that, I'm becoming increasingly frustrated that I still do not have the equipment I need to do my job and therefore I need you to speak to the suppliers to obtain a firm commitment as to a delivery date.'

'I found our conversation this morning really valuable as you seemed very keen to understand the difficulties I have lip reading people when everyone in the meeting is talking at once. Thank you for taking on board my suggestions. Having said that, with the current conversation everybody has started to talk all at once again and I cannot follow what is being said. I really need you all to talk one at a time please so that I can listen to the conversation and take an active part in it.'

'I really appreciate you wanting to help me across the street. Thanks for asking. However, I like doing things for myself and I therefore need to cross on my own please.'

Every time I gave Paul another scenario or example he was able to use his ten words to deal with it. He conceded that these ten words would not always work in helping me to get what I needed. But by using them I had a structure for the conversation and this built my confidence in dealing with scenarios that either I had never tackled before, or that I had tackled but not got the result I really needed.

Paul drew things to a close. 'I really enjoyed meeting you Chris and thank you for coming. It was great for me to have the opportunity to explore these concepts again. I will be really disappointed though if you do nothing with these ideas as I know that they will help you and therefore I want you to practise them and you will see a real difference to the impact you have and also to your confidence.'

There were his ten words again and I could see how powerful they were. I assured him that the conversation had been invigorating and challenging and that I was convinced the concepts he'd shared would help me move on.

I came away from Paul's session feeling so empowered it was untrue. I practised using the ten word structure for the next few days in all sorts of scenarios, regularly changing my words so that I did not come across like a parrot using a script. I used it in a shop to say what I was not happy with and what I needed them to do differently to correct their mistake and I did so with appropriate words, music and dance so they understood my message but I was not aggressive.

I spoke to some local children, using this approach, to tell them how I felt about them playing football near the windows of my house. They were okay about moving on because I showed them that I understood their agenda and recognised their desire to play.

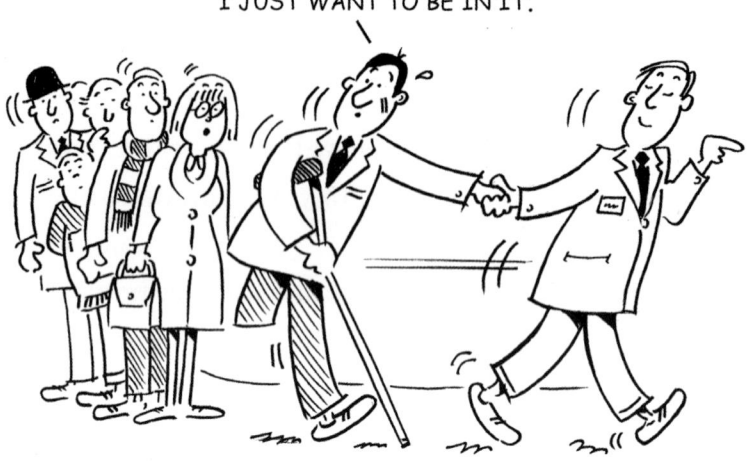

I first considered how useful this approach was and thought that if only I had known about it years before I would have got so much more of my own way. I then thought again and understood how selfish that initial thought was and realised that actually if we all talked to each other in this way then we would all get along better. Be honest and clear about your own agenda at the same time as really showing that you have understood, recognised and valued the other person's agenda. If you don't recognise theirs, why should they recognise yours?

For the next week, I became more aware of what other people were saying and how people's written and spoken language was absolutely littered with diluting words and phrases. I lost count of how many times I heard phrases like, 'If it's ok with you' or 'I could do with' or 'I would like to' or 'It would be nice if' or 'I'm quite happy' or 'maybe, possibly and probably' and I saw the effect they all had was to dilute the message.

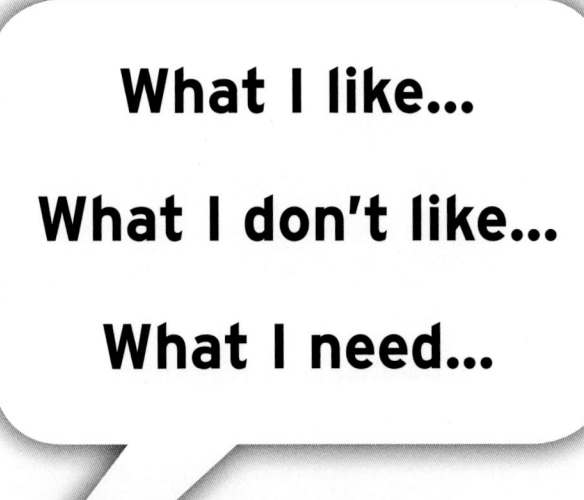

> What I like…
>
> What I don't like…
>
> What I need…

6 Me

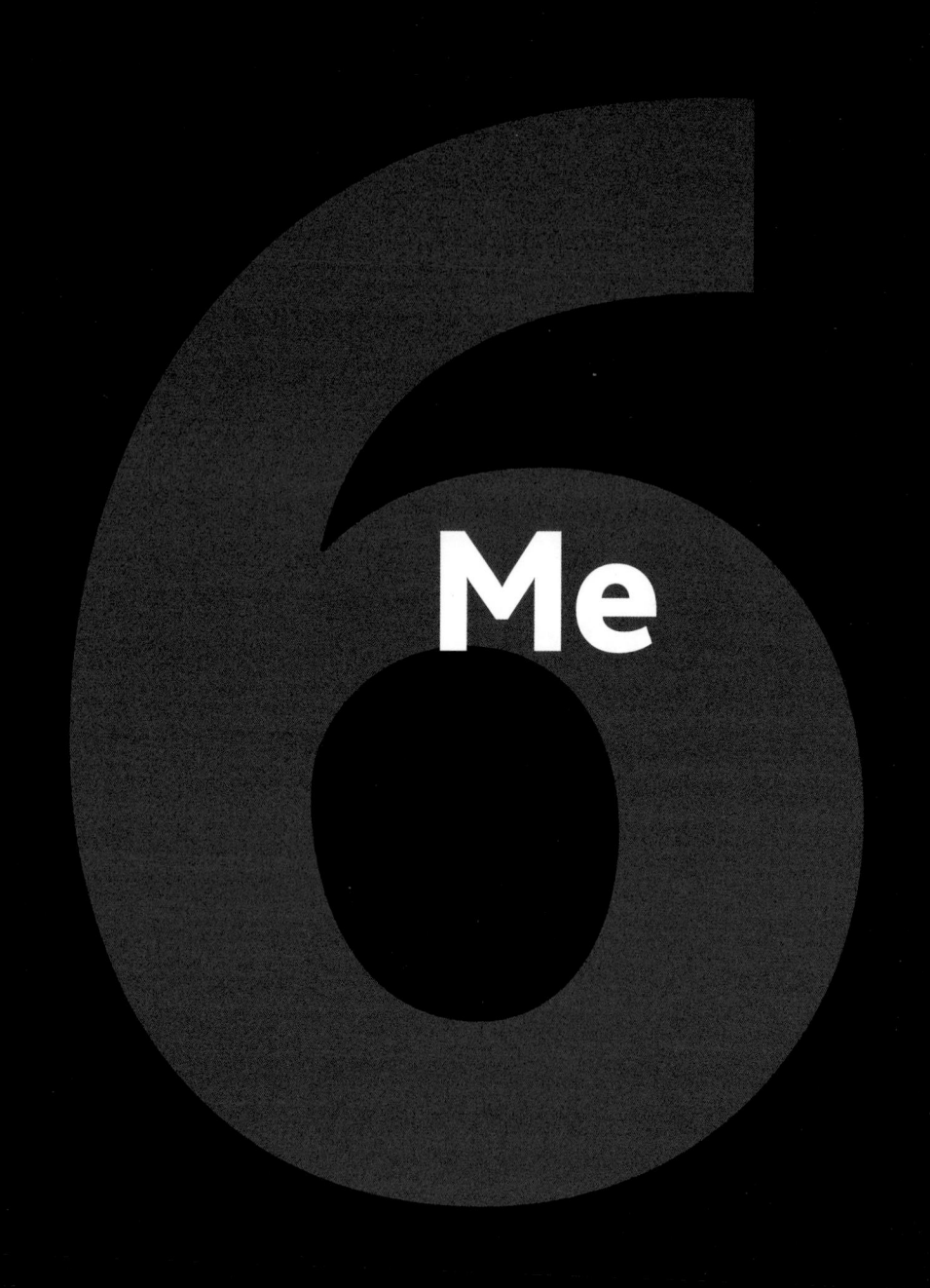

I had absorbed so much by meeting Dawn's disabled colleagues. I had also learnt other skills that were completely unexpected.

I was keen to meet up with Dawn again to thank her for helping to change my life and to see what she thought might be next for me.

We had arranged to meet in a small coffee shop and despite the cold and wet weather, I felt incredibly upbeat and positive. The shop was busy with lots of customers chatting to each other but I was so engrossed in our own conversation that I didn't notice anyone else.

Once we'd found a table and I'd ordered some drinks I launched into telling Dawn how much I wanted to thank her for arranging for me to meet her extraordinary and helpful colleagues. I had discovered so much and it had really helped me to see myself and the world in a different way. I also said that not only had I learnt a huge amount, I had also *un*learned a great deal that had enabled me to move forward.

'I'm so pleased,' replied Dawn. 'I knew you would benefit from meeting them. So tell me exactly what you feel you've learnt.'

I began with my first session with George. He had helped me to understand the importance of language. If I described myself as 'suffering' or a 'victim' or 'having a problem' then other people would see me that way so I had to use positive language and then people would treat me more positively. George also reminded me of the bereavement process and its relevance to those people who joined the disability club at some point in their lives. They grieved for their loss and it was important to work through that process and start to become more positive about themselves and their situation, whatever the problems or condition they now had.

Next there was Angela who had helped me to understand how crucial it was to talk appropriately about your impairment and its impact on those around you. Her phrases 'everybody is normal', and 'it's normal to be different' had made a real impact on me. Even though society has various views of 'different', if you change the context then you change the view.

I had learnt about the various models of disability from Jan – the medical and charity models – and how they have been used, intentionally and unintentionally, to help us but that they haven't always done this. The social model is the most powerful and effective because it positions us as having challenges rather than being the problem; it is the way society ignores or excludes that really disables us.

Finally, Paul had helped me to pull it all together and to do something with all this knowledge. He had helped me to understand the principles of words, music and dance and how to become more assertive in asking for what I needed. Alternatively, when I didn't need their help, I would need to tell the person in an appropriate and positive way.

I then asked Dawn, 'Tell me, how did you get to work with these people?'

'Well I am what some might call a carer,' she replied. 'My

partner has an impairment and I wanted to know how I could help him and myself. We knew George as a friend and I asked him to help me. He works for an organisation run by people with impairments that provides support to disabled people and their families. He introduced me to the same people that you met and they went through the same principles with me as they did with you. I remember at the time that I was getting annoyed, for instance, that people would ask me if my partner was ok. I would say, 'Why don't you ask him? He's perfectly capable of answering you!' I was annoyed that as a mum it was fine for me to work part-time three days a week but when my partner asked to adjust his hours to help him better manage his disability that was difficult. The world around him was treating him differently just because he now had an impairment.'

Dawn went on to say that her partner was also disabling himself by, for instance, not asking others for help when clearly it would have been the best thing to do. 'When we went shopping he insisted on walking to get around the shops saying, "this thing isn't going to beat me". I quite understood that this was his way of trying to stay independent, but truthfully it completely wore him out and then he had no energy for anything else. It made it more difficult to do the shopping. His wish to be seen as 'normal' meant he would not use a wheelchair or ask for help when carrying things upstairs or any distance. The whole thing was really difficult.'

I was engrossed in her story as I considered that it must be the same story for so many other people in similar situations.

Dawn continued. 'I wrestled with how I should act as a carer. Should I just help or make decisions? I could do things and make decisions for him and that made things so much easier. But I came to realise that they made things easier for me. I needed to help him with the things he couldn't do and let him do the things he could do, however difficult or time consuming they were. For his part he needed to manage his impairment more effectively so that using a wheelchair could be viewed as no different to using a car; it sometimes makes life easier even if it might be perceived as lazy!'

She went on to explain that she was also going through her own bereavement process in relation to her partner's disability. She had gone through the shock and denial stages followed by the anger, frustration and guilt, even though it was her partner who had the impairment, not her. It was similar to me going through these stages when my friends had died.

She had considered the appropriate sharing and disclosure element very carefully as her partner's impairment was not visible at first but still had an impact on their ability to do certain things.

'In the end,' she added, 'with the help of the disabled people you met he learnt to manage his condition despite it being progressive and so we both have to go through the bereavement curve again and again for each stage of the condition. He explored really helpful ideas like putting together a one-page document that described his impairment, its impact – what he was able to do and not able to do – and then finally what he wanted from other people. He used to give it out at work to his managers and colleagues and customers so that he was managing the impact of his impairment on them. It was very liberating I can tell you, but it was only after speaking with disabled colleagues that we thought of doing that. So there you are,' Dawn finished. 'The journey continues and I know that the people we've both met will provide support as best they can as and when we need it. So please do stay in touch. You have my contact details.'

I thanked Dawn for everything and assured her that I would call her if I needed to and she should feel she could do the same with me.

We finished our drinks and I left the coffee shop reflecting on what Dawn and her partner were dealing with every day of their lives: ordinary people doing ordinary things but with an extraordinary perspective.

As I travelled home I contemplated once again the journey I had made and the distance still to cover. Clearly we are all dealt different cards in our lives. Sometimes we get good hands, sometimes not. It's not the hand that you are dealt though; it's the way that you play it that matters.

I realised that in a race I might be last but I am not a loser if I apply these principles and keep learning to apply them better.

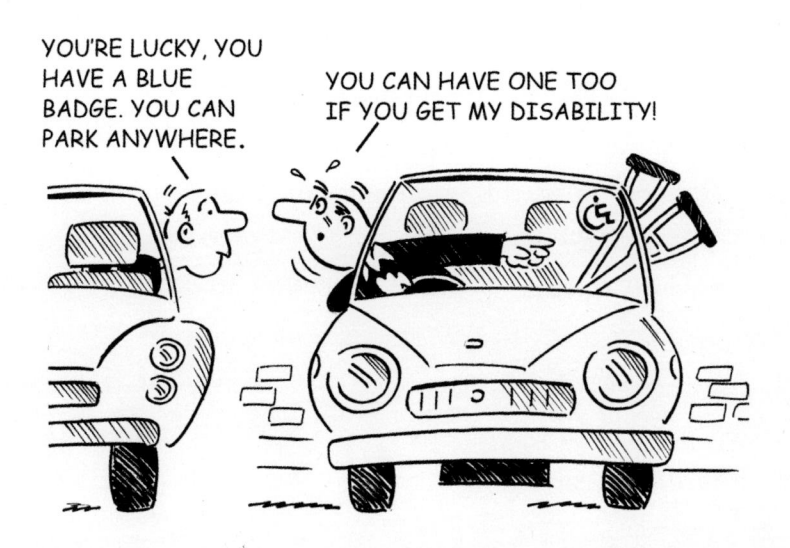

7 You

So why have I told you my story?

Well I guess that depends on why you are reading this.

I still meet people with impairments who ask: 'Why me? Why did this happen to me? What did I do to deserve this?' The responses are many and varied and usually unhelpful. 'To remind the rest of us how lucky we are,' or, 'Why not you? – Would you wish this on somebody else? Maybe you're strong enough to deal with it.'

The absolute fact is most of us are born without impairments but the majority of us will acquire one before we depart this life. So we should see its onset as part of being alive and being human – yet another challenging human difference. By applying a social model approach, we understand that our disability stems from the attitudes of others or the physical barriers that exclude us. While we may not be able to 'fix' the impairment, we can certainly do something about the things that disable us.

If you have an impairment and feel that you are being disabled by it, then I hope that by sharing my story I have given you some new ideas with which to tackle the world in a positive way. People have asked me whether they are disabled enough to use these ideas and my answer is that you are never 'sort of' pregnant – you either are pregnant or you're not. Therefore, if you have an impairment and are being disabled either because of the limitations of your own self-belief or because of the behaviours and attitudes of others then these ideas and tools are for you.

We don't have 'special needs'. Every one of us living on this planet is special. We just have 'additional needs' and we have the right to have these needs met in order for us to contribute and add value.

Remember that you are learning things as a result of your impairment that others who are not disabled are not learning – yet.

I wanted you to know what I have learnt and have had

to unlearn to help me to focus on managing my disability rather than merely coping with my impairment. I know now that I need to take control and manage other people in a positive way so they feel more comfortable in dealing with me and my impairment. I will reap what I sow but the harvest will be different now.

Needless to say I now never apologise for being disabled – why should I?

I never put myself down in order to make other people more comfortable – why should I? I still use humour an awful lot, however, I don't use it to poke fun at my situation. I may be funny but I am not the joke.

In this way, I still have the condition I have but I have reduced my disability.

In essence I have stopped pretending to be normal because I am as normal as everyone else. We are all normal because we are all different.

George's comment, 'I am who I am as a result of my impairment not in spite of it,' has made me think deeply. I feel whatever I want to feel about the impairment I have, it is now a part of me; part of who I am for the remainder of my life – I cannot deny or ignore that.

The main reason for sharing my story is to help you, the reader, whether you are someone with an impairment or supporting somebody with one, or whether you are someone who is interested in the area of disability and how to view it effectively.

I am delighted that you have read this book (what I like); although I would be really disappointed if you did nothing with what I have shared with you (what I don't like);
and so I need you to use it to help yourself and others learn to live with disability by using the ideas I have presented to you.

After all barriers that disable us will remain a part of the human story of our future if we don't do something differently.

Good luck!

Are you disabled by other people's perceptions of you **or by your own perceptions of you?**

We can't cure your impairment but **we can do something about your disability**.

What they say about this book

"Normality is that boring space between everything that is exciting and exceptional but some disabled people think it is the safe space they should occupy. This book shows disabled people need to be themselves and not follow the yellow brick road to "Normality". Through a number of conversations with disabled people Chris, who has a recently acquired impairment, is challenged on why he tries to appear normal. Just as Tressell's "The Ragged Trousered Philanthropist" explained socialism clearer than Karl Marx ever achieved, this book explains the social and medical models of disability through every-day conversations that turn complex ideas on impairment and disability into common sense that we can all understand. Well worth reading!"
Sir Bert Massie CBE

"Whether you acquire an impairment during your lifetime or grow up with one, it is all too easy to absorb the norms and attitudes of the culture around you and become disabled by them. That makes it all the harder to deal with the other barriers that disable. I was privileged to have a sister, and disabled friends, who taught me different! For those many disabled people who are not so privileged and who have to deal with the internalised oppression this

creates by themselves, this book cuts through those norms and attitudes in a refreshing and simple way. I hope that it will start many people on the journey to an empowered life where they no longer see themselves as 'the problem', but understand where the real problems lie so they can deal with them."
Alice Maynard, Director, Future Inclusion

"This book should be read by any professional that works either directly or on the fringes with disabled people from, doctors, nurses, social workers, benefits advisors etc. In fact it should be read by everyone including children in school as it offers great insight into the lives of disabled people and how we wish to be treated."
Julie Fernandez Actress, Producer and Disability Rights Campaigner

"This book is bursting with great ideas based on a unique wealth of personal experience of both the reality of disability and the reality of work - employers wanting to realise the potential of every employee should ensure copies are readily and widely available."
Susan Scott Parker OBE, CEO Business Disability Forum.

"I think the book will be extremely valuable in stimulating discussion not solely by people with disabilities and their families but the wider community."
The Right Honourable David Blunkett, MP.

"Phil Friend and Dave Rees have been making a positive difference to the lives and careers of disabled employees for over ten years. Their inspirational approach deserves a far bigger audience so I'm delighted to endorse this book. I really believe it will help disabled people overcome the barriers too many of them still face to success and self-fulfilment"
Tim Taylor, Manager, Diversity & Inclusion, Lloyds Banking Group.

"If you or someone you know wants to understand disability better, how it fits in society today, this is a great place to start. Using accessible language and with a respectful nod to Socratic dialogue, the narrative follows the enlightenment of the main character who begins to make sense of how their behaviour and thinking, and that of those around them, can have a greater impact on their life than their 'disability'. You'll still be the same person after reading this, but how you see yourself or others with a disability is likely

to have shifted. It's one of those books that needs to be written, needs to exist, so everyone can understand a bit more about what disability is and what it isn't."
Simon Minty, Director, Sminty Ltd.

Acknowledgements

Anyone who has ever written a book knows just how much you come to rely on the support and encouragement of lots of different people. Some are close friends and family, some are people who you meet along the way and some are those who said something that got you thinking. We are indebted to all of them but some deserve a special mention.

First we say thank you to both our families, specifically Sue, Carole and Maddi for their enthusiasm, encouragement, suggestions and patience. They were also involved in the proof reading and critiquing of the book as were Giles Cockman, Geoff Adam-Spink, Simon Minty, Kate Nash, Emma Dixon, Kevin Fitzpatrick, and Alice Maynard. Thanks also to Colin Davidson for the cartoons.

We are truly indebted to Jane Cordell and Peter Dupont for their support, guidance, proof reading, ideas, editing, contacts and all manner of hints and tips which you need to know when publishing a book. Their belief in the messages and also in us was a hugely important factor in this book seeing the light of day. Roy Williams also provided valuable advice and ideas as to how the book should look.

A special mention for Baroness Tanni Grey Thompson

who took time out from an incredibly busy work schedule to write the Foreword for the book. Thank you also to all those who have provided quotes and opinions that confirmed to us that this book had value.

There are others we should like to thank who have provided us with invaluable support and ideas throughout the years, specifically Andrew Wakelin, Tim Taylor, Judith Langley, John Spence and Val Thorpe. It is also important not to forget the individual who first asked the question of Phil – why are you pretending to be normal? We wish we knew her name. She is probably unaware of the impact she had and she needs to know the profound effect that question had all those years ago. Many thanks.

Finally our biggest thanks go to all those many, many wonderful inspirational people who we have met as part of our Career Development and Personal Development Programmes. Without their belief in our messages and the constant feedback they provided this book would never have been written.

Thank You!
Phil and Dave

The authors

Phil Friend

Phil was born in London and contracted polio in 1949.

As a wheelchair user he worked in social work until the late 1980's but since setting up his business he has focussed on disability in the workplace. He has been engaged by some of the UK's major corporations and public sector organisations and has had a significant influence on how organisations manage disability in the workplace.

He is married to Sue, lives in Hertfordshire and has four children and three grandchildren.

Dave Rees

Dave has spent 20 years training and developing people in enhancing their communication and influencing skills in the workplace. He is a Chartered Manager with the Chartered Management Institute and supports managers to understand what impact they have and how they can improve their effectiveness in leadership skills.

Along with Phil he designed and has delivered the Personal and Career Development Programmes for Disabled Staff since 2001.

He was born in Shropshire, is married to Carole, has a daughter and lives in South Wales.